Rethinking ADHD

Rethinking ADHD

Integrated approaches to helping children at home and at school

16080/

Ruth Schmidt Neven, Vicki Anderson and Tim Godber

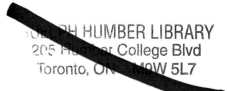
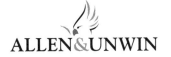

ALLEN&UNWIN

First published in 2002 by
Allen & Unwin
83 Alexander Street
Crows Nest NSW 2065
Australia
Phone: (61 2) 8425 0100
Fax: (61 2) 9906 2218
Email: info@allenandunwin.com
Web: www.allenandunwin.com

National Library of Australia
Cataloguing-in-Publication entry:

Neven, Ruth Schmidt.
 Rethinking ADHD: integrated approaches to helping children
 at home and at school.

 Bibliography.
 Includes index.
 ISBN 1 86508 816 1.

 1. Attention-deficit hyperactivity disorder. 2. Behavioral
 assessment of children. I. Anderson, Vicki A. II. Godber,
 Tim. III. Title.

618.928589

Typeset by Midland Typesetters
Printed by Southwood Press

10 9 8 7 6 5 4 3 2 1

Contents

About the authors

Ruth Schmidt Neven is a child and adult psychotherapist who trained at the Tavistock Clinic in England. With over 30 years' experience of work with children, parents and adolescents, she is committed to promoting knowledge and understanding about child and family development in the broader community. She has been a pioneer in the field of parent education in the United Kingdom, setting up the national organisation Exploring Parenthood. She came to Australia in 1989 to take up the first position of Chief Psychotherapist at the Royal Children's Hospital in Melbourne, a post she held until 1994. Ruth is currently the director of the Centre for Child and Family Development, which offers counselling and psychotherapy to children and families, as well as professional training courses. Ruth writes and lectures extensively on all aspects of child development and parenting in Australia and overseas. She has provided training and consultancy to government and non-government agencies. She has written two books, *Exploring Parenthood* and *Emotional Milestones: From Birth to Adulthood*, both published by the Australian Council for Educational Research. She is currently engaged in research on how professionals construct the mental health problems of children and families.

Vicki Anderson, PhD, is a paediatric neuropsychologist of some twenty years' experience who currently holds positions as a Senior Lecturer, Department of Psychology, University of Melbourne, and Senior Research & Clinical Neuropsychologist, Royal Children's

Hospital, Melbourne. She started her career at the Royal Children's Hospital, where she worked as a clinician and then Coordinator of Neuropsychology Services, until taking up a lectureship at the University of Melbourne. Her interests are in disorders of childhood that impact on the central nervous system, including both developmental and acquired disorders. She has published over 40 papers in this field and has attracted over one million dollars in research funding. Her research group has recently established the Centre for Child Neuropsychological Studies (CNS) at the Royal Children's Hospital.

Tim Godber lectures in psychological assessment and health psychology at La Trobe University in the Bachelor of Public Health, Bachelor of Pharmacy and Bachelor of Behavioural Science degree programs. He is a psychologist and teacher with extensive experience working with children and parents in Australia and overseas. His research career began at the Royal Children's Hospital with a study of the cognitive effects of cranial irradiation and his interests now focus on preventive mental health, the impact of developmental disability on family functioning and the diagnostic issues associated with the use of paediatric intelligence tests.

1

Rethinking ADHD:
An illness of our time

The past ten to fifteen years have seen significant changes in the way in which children's behaviour problems have been described and diagnosed. These changes have been particularly striking in North America where, according to Barkley (1998a), 3–5 per cent of the school-age population has been prescribed psychostimulant drugs. Australia and the United Kingdom have also experienced dramatic increases in the numbers of children and adolescents diagnosed with attention deficit disorder (ADD) or attention deficit hyperactivity disorder (ADHD). In Australia for example, there has been a twentyfold increase in prescription rates for these drugs since 1990 and current figures indicate that more than 300 000 prescriptions are issued annually (Mackey & Kopras, 2001). In North America the increase in rates of diagnosis for ADHD and drug prescriptions has been so rapid that the statistics are considered to be obsolete by the time they are published in scientific journals (McCubbin & Cohen, 1999).

What is ADHD? How the problem is currently presented

The fourth edition of the Diagnostic and Statistical Manual of Mental Disorders (DSM-IV), published by the American Psychiatric Association and regarded as the standard internationally recognised manual of criteria for the assessment and diagnosis of mental disorder, identifies the three core manifestations of ADHD as

Inattention, Hyperactivity and Impulsiveness. In order for this diagnosis to take place, six or more symptoms related to each of these categories need to have been present for at least six months. The symptoms related to attentional problems include behaviours such as difficulty in maintaining attention, inability to listen and carry out instructions, difficulty in organising tasks, distractibility and forgetfulness. The symptoms related to hyperactivity–impulsivity include fidgetiness, excessive activity and difficulty in sustaining play. In addition the criteria specify that some impairment must be present in two or more settings, such as home and school, and that there must be clinically significant impairment in social, academic or occupational functioning. The presence of some of these symptoms before the age of seven is also seen as significant for the diagnosis (see Appendix 1).

The DSM-IV classification further allows for what is known as a differential diagnosis. This means that subgroups can be identified within these broader categories. For example, some children might meet the criteria for attention problems but not hyperactive–impulsive problems. They would therefore be diagnosed as ADHD predominantly inattentive type. In other children where attentional problems do not appear to be significant but where there are behavioural difficulties, a diagnosis of ADHD predominantly hyperactive/impulsive type can be made.

A brief history of ADHD

The earliest identification of attentional problems in children was made by the paediatrician Frederick Still, in 1902, in an article published in the *Lancet*. Still identified a group of children displaying an inability for sustained attention combined with restlessness and fidgetiness. At the time, Still argued that these behaviours had a biological origin. The British Psychological Society report on attention deficit hyperactivity disorder (BPS, 1996) provides an excellent overview of the difficulties associated with subsequent and ongoing attempts to find conclusive evidence of biological markers for hyperactivity and behavioural problems as well as the identification of specific categories of children who display these problems. The report describes how the history of ADHD was linked to the chance discovery by Bradley (1937) in the United States that the psychostimulant amphetamine could reduce levels of hyperactivity and behavioural problems. The 1950s and 1960s saw the strengthening of the belief in the specific identification of children with hyperactivity and in the disorder's biological origins. This led to the introduction of terms such as minimal brain damage and minimal brain dysfunction applied to children who often exhibited a wide range of behavioural and learning problems. As the BPS report points out, the term minimal brain dysfunction eventually became a 'catch-all' concept, even for children who showed no signs of neurological dysfunction.

Subsequent attempts at reformulating the problem focused increasingly on the observation of the behaviour of overactive children, particularly with regard to their capacity for attention. The emergence of ADHD as a diagnostic category owes much to the conviction of researchers in the field that attention and not hyper-activity is the core factor that distinguishes these children from children who may be simply difficult and disruptive. In particular the research of Douglas (1972), which found that hyperactive children performed badly on standardised tests of attention, led to the estab-lishment of attention deficit disorder as a category in the third edition of the *Diagnostic and Statistical Manual of Mental Disorders* (DSM-III) published by the American Psychiatric Association (1980).

As the BPS report states, in this first phase of the emergence of the concept of ADHD, there was a shift in emphasis from aetiology (the cause of a medical condition) to behavioural expression. This meant that a diagnosis of ADD or ADHD was made on the basis of the observation of children's actual behaviour. This shift in emphasis towards the behaviour of the child has led to the view that the symptoms have *become* the syndrome (Reid, 1995, cited in the BPS report, p. 14).

The primacy of the medical model: Implications for understanding ADHD

The formal diagnosis of ADD and ADHD is one that can only be made by medical practitioners who are also in a position to prescribe drugs to alleviate or contain the symptoms. This has had important implications, not only for the way in which ADD and ADHD have been perceived and described, but also for the consid-erable increase in drug prescriptions. The medical model rests on a fundamental assumption about the presence or absence of an illness, disease or malfunction. It is a model that is entirely focused on the individual's physical status and on physiological processes within the body that can be directly observed and measured. As such, the medical model with its exclusive focus on disease operates within very narrow parameters. It does not take into account, for example, the often subtle and complex interrelationship between mind and body and the impact that emotional and indeed social experience can have on physical health and functioning.

In this book we question some of the commonly held views about ADHD—in particular, the at times strongly held belief that it is a discrete and exclusively medical condition as described above. A purely medical approach positions the problem firmly within the child and apparently relieves the parents and family of a sense of guilt or blame. As we discuss in this book, we believe that this is a simplistic response that misrepresents the context of the problem, namely the complex interrelationship between the child (both psychological and physical aspects), the child's parents and family relationships, and the broader community. Labelling ADHD as a disease shuts out the consideration of a broader context and might lead to the isolation of the child, to the disempowerment of parents and ultimately to a misdirected treatment.

As the British Psychological Society report concludes, we should be cautious about unquestioningly accepting a diagnosis of ADHD as a mental disorder for large groups of children whose difficulties might be due to a multiplicity of factors. We also need to recognise the limitations of studies purporting to provide absolute biological or psychological markers for the problem. Most importantly, the report suggests we need to develop environmental as well as individual approaches to intervention and encourage greater cooperation between all the professionals involved in the life of the child.

The demographics of diagnosis

The complexities in the assessment and diagnosis of ADHD are exemplified in the wide variations reported in relation to gender, socioeconomic status and geography. For example:

- A far higher proportion of boys are diagnosed with ADHD, than girls. While estimates vary according to how the data is collected, current estimates suggest that between three and six males are diagnosed for every one female (Barkley, 1990; Szatmari, Offord & Boyle, 1989). According to the Australian National Health and Medical Research Council (1997), in all age groups estimates of the male to female ratio for ADHD range from 4:1 to 9:1.

- The socioeconomic status of the family appears to play a part in the decision making about the diagnosis. Anecdotal evidence from professionals suggests that a greater proportion of children from low socioeconomic backgrounds are diagnosed with the condition than children from more middle-class backgrounds (Prosser, 1997).
- Similarly, anecdotal evidence suggests that a disproportionately high number of children in various forms of institutional care are regularly prescribed medication.
- Where the child lives appears to be a factor in the diagnosis of ADHD. In Australia, one study found that five times as many families have their child receive a diagnosis of ADHD in New South Wales than in the neighbouring state of Victoria (Mellor, Storer & Brown, 1996). More recent analysis has uncovered an even wider disparity in the prescription of medication for children with ADHD (Mackey & Kopras, 2001). Western Australia, with one of the smallest populations in Australia, has the highest prescription rate, more than six times the rate per person in Victoria. While some might argue that this indicates higher diagnostic skills among some medical practitioners, this is not a view that is universally shared. In the United States, rates of diagnosis of ADHD also vary widely between different states (Mackey & Kopras, 2001).
- It has been found that small numbers of medical practitioners in certain areas can be responsible for high prescription rates. For example, research in this area in Adelaide in South Australia found that five prescribers were responsible for 61 per cent of patients (Prosser & Reid, 1999).

These demographic factors may indicate not so much that we have hard evidence that these groups present with a higher incidence of ADHD, but rather that we may be able to build up a picture of how and why these children receive such a diagnosis in the first place. In other words, this information might tell us more about the current diagnostic practice of the practitioners who carry out the diagnosis and the circumstances surrounding the diagnosis than about the children themselves.

As the health commentator Dr Norman Swan states:

As soon as you see variations like that in medicine and health, it's usually the fact that there's non-evidence-based treatment going on, that there's opinion-based treatment going on. (ABC Radio, *The Health Report*, 23 October 2000)

ADHD—an illness of our time?

We believe that it is particularly significant that ADHD has moved into such prominence at the present time. One way of understanding this is to recognise that it has in effect become 'the illness of our time' and that the timing and appearance of this diagnosis might owe very little to chance. Social researcher Hugh Mackay, writing in Melbourne's *Age* (1999) of 'Childhood's Brave New World', describes the unprecedented changes taking place in child-rearing and in the daily arrangements being made for children as representing 'a vast social experiment', the results of which will only become known in subsequent generations. Mackay refers to parents wondering 'whether they are teaching their children, from too early an age, to juggle time; whether there is a danger of over-stimulation in all this frenetic activity that might lead to heightened anxiety, depression or other disorders in the young'.

The unprecedented social changes in family and community life have an impact on how we view child development and the problems of childhood. Clinical experience and research (Billington, 1996; Breggin, 1994, 1999) suggest that there is an increasing tendency for child and family mental health professionals to fragment and compartmentalise the problems of the children and parents they are trying to help. This tendency towards fragmentation leads professionals and services to address the child's problem in an instrumental manner, outside of the child or adolescent's developmental, interpersonal, family and social experience. In this context ADHD might become a *disposal diagnosis*. An example is the tendency for some professionals to refer to a child as if 'he *is* ADD or ADHD'. The use of language in this manner depersonalises the child and turns the subject—the child, into the object. The tendency towards fragmentation might also go some way to explaining the relief that many parents feel when a medical diagnosis of ADD or ADHD is made about their child, since this limits the need for any broader enquiry into family life and interpersonal relationships.

In this book, we argue that the diagnostic category of ADHD covers a wide range of symptoms with many underlying causes. While we maintain that for a subgroup of children these symptoms might indicate the presence of neurological factors, that is factors relating to the nervous system and disorders thereof, for many others the rush to diagnosis reflects primarily psychosocial considerations. We are nevertheless concerned that many children will not be adequately treated for the problems they have. It has, for example, long been acknowledged by prominent researchers in the field that many of the symptoms described as typical of ADHD are in fact also symptoms of other problems. In the UK, Rutter (1982) has pointed out that 'there is no empirical support for a unitary concept of Attention Deficit which is common to many disorders'. We thus support the view that ADHD is an umbrella term that covers a variety of disturbances and encompasses a diverse group of children.

An alternative view of ADHD: Parent and child relationships

We believe that the term ADHD, rather than being used to describe a range of behaviours of a child, in fact epitomises the idea of 'an illness of our time', where attention is perceived solely as a cognitive function of the brain rather than as a complex and multi-dimensional activity that emerges out of a relational process between children, parents and caregivers. While there are powerful maturational and biological processes involved in the rapidly increasing attentional abilities of children as they develop, it is the parent–child relationship that is of equal importance for *the emergence of a mind and the capacity for thought*—a capacity that includes emotional as well as intellectual competence. Thus we believe that it is the appropriate *interaction* between biological, psychological and emotional experience that sets the scene for healthy development.

At a time when parenting is receiving so much publicity and the parenting field is almost akin to an industry, the surprising paradox is that we remain so much in the dark about our understanding of the inner world of the child. Our greater understanding of the needs of parents does not appear to have translated into greater knowledge of what children need in order to flourish and grow. The proliferation of ADHD diagnoses would appear to be a particularly potent example of this state of affairs.

Dramatic reductions in the average number of children within each family, together with the more sharply defined notions of 'success' and expectations to conform, which are now prevalent in our society, mean that there is an increasing emphasis on children as the visible outcomes of *parenting* (note the transformation of a noun into an active verb). The pressure on children to perform and to succeed has percolated down into the primary school and kindergarten with many parents now seeing 'average' as barely acceptable and 'delayed' as prima facie evidence of disease. It would be surprising if a situation as volatile as this did not contribute to the epidemic of ADHD 'cases' that has occurred in Western countries, compounded as it is by the confused signals sent by the professionals involved in the debate and the misgivings felt by many about the pharmaceutical solutions increasingly being sought.

To complicate matters, much of the literature and discourse concerned with child-rearing today is resonant with language that conjures up the tactics of the boardroom and the battlefield rather than ideas that are useful for an understanding of children and their behaviour. Parents are encouraged to 'tame' their children, to find 'strategies' for managing their behaviour and indeed to be critical of the 'attention-seeking child'. Some of the ideas of economic rationalism have also managed to find their way into this discourse with its focus on 'controlled crying', even 'controlled comforting' as though relational experience is a commodity, with finite inputs of time and energy, that must be strictly accounted for. While these are responses that are understandable in anxious parents, the approaches themselves provide little evidence that they address the underlying cause of the problem for children.

One way of trying to make sense of this plethora of information and advice is to view it as an attempt to control the painful and difficult events of everyday life. The sense of chaos engendered by overactive, inattentive children might indeed lead parents and professionals to run for cover behind narrow diagnostic categories and even narrower options for treatment. Such a strategy might prevail even when it ultimately compounds the problem and sells children short.

In this book we consider the attentional requirements of *all* children and how the recommendations we make for the ADHD group can be applied to the wider population. This view enables us to place ADHD within the context of a *broader child and family public mental health domain*. Here we consider the interface between the individual child's problem and the emotional, social, economic and cultural factors that all play a part in 'creating' the behaviour.

We also try to forge what we hope are more creative links between an understanding of the physical aspects of *brain* activity associated with attentional processes and the psychological development of the *mind*, and the child's capacity for thought. Central to our argument is a recognition that the attachment of infants and young children to their caregivers forms the emotional foundation for life and in fact interacts with neurological functioning, thus contributing to the child's capacity for learning, social interaction and sense of self.

While this interaction operates effectively in the majority of children and families, there are extreme situations where attachment is impaired or lost through neglect, depression or separation so that the child experiences a 'rupture' that has implications for all aspects of growth and development. Infants and young children whose primary caregiver is unavailable to them owing to illness, depression, loss or trauma lose the critical *organising–containing function*, which is an essential part of this relational experience. The parent or caregiver helps to give meaning to the child's experience so that the organising–containing function of the caregiver operates *par excellence* on the boundary of emotional and cognitive functioning.

The concept of self-regulation: Linking the brain and the mind

Self-regulation, arising as it does from our understanding of the various autonomic systems within the body that regulate the function of the heart, lungs, brain and digestion, proves to be a particularly fruitful construct when we consider the link between the structural aspects of brain function and the development of personality. As Siegel (2001) states, the essence of the function of the mind (which he sees as patterns of the flow of energy and information) is a product of neurophysiology as well as interpersonal interaction. This, Siegel believes, leads us to an exciting convergence of findings from neuroscience as well as from the behavioural sciences, in particular our understanding of child development.

In this book, and consistent with others in the field (Barkley, 1997a, 1998a), we argue that many of the 'hyperactive' type symptoms generally associated with ADHD can be viewed as problems associated with disturbances in the capacity for self-regulation. From a neuropsychological perspective the difficulties experienced by some children diagnosed with ADHD might be accounted for by abnormalities in the areas of the brain responsible for developing strategies, monitoring their implementation and making suitable adjustments in response to feedback about performance. From the psychodynamic perspective on child development, the capacity for self-regulation arises out of the earliest relationship between the infant and their caregivers, and is by its very nature 'psychosomatic' in that it operates on the boundary of the physical and the emotional. We will present recent evidence in support of the contention that these early relationships may actually alter brain physiology and function. This research will be used to further demonstrate the points of contact between neuropsychological, developmental and emotional considerations in conceptualising ADHD.

A new paradigm

If we are to place the exploration of ADHD within the broader context of the child and family public health domain, then it forces us to adopt a new model of thinking—a new paradigm, one that enables us to integrate our knowledge of the physical workings of the brain with our understanding of the psychological and emotional development of the mind.

On looking back over the past century, it would be fair to say that the tendency within the sciences has been towards an ever-increasing specialisation. This has led to a decrease in communication between disciplines, and in some cases even within disciplines. The fragmentation that has taken place within psychology is a good example of this process. For example, there has been little dialogue between those practitioners trained in the field of neuropsychology and those trained in the field of psychotherapy, often to the detriment of the people they are trying to help.

However, as we begin a new century there is a growing awareness of the need to extend our thinking, to explore new paradigms and to develop a greater potential for synthesis and for the identification of essential interrelationships between and within systems.

This leads us to see what Siegel (2001) calls a 'unity of knowledge' or what Wilson (1998) has described as 'consilience'. The complex presentation of ADHD lends itself particularly well to an exploration that can move beyond the linear thinking of symptom and syndrome, allowing us to look for patterns of interrelationship within a broader context. It is for this reason that we introduce an attempted integration of neuropsychological and psychodynamic approaches to understanding ADHD, a condition that appears to operate on the boundary between brain function (the realm of neuropsychology and neurology) and the child's emotional and social relationships within the family and the outside world (explored in the psychodynamic approach).

This book represents an extension of the collaborative work carried out in our ADHD training workshops. These workshops have been run mainly for professionals but also for parents. The one-day sessions for professionals working in social work, paediatrics, psychology, teaching, nursing, early childhood, general medical practice and community work brought home to us the realisation that an understanding of the needs of children and adolescents who present with ADHD, must inevitably relate to an understanding of the needs of *all* children and young people. Indeed our collaborative effort has led us to a position that emphasises that an understanding of ADHD and a focus on prevention are inextricable. Thus, as we explain in the following chapters, broadening the paradigm has the potential to extend prevention into the important realm of public health.

The workshops we have run on ADHD are an example of broadening the paradigm. They have created opportunities for professionals from different disciplines to talk to each other. This has led to the workshop itself becoming a learning environment, which widens the discourse about the origins of the problem and enables professionals to think differently and creatively about potential solutions. Two main conclusions have emerged from these multidisciplinary workshops: the first is that the segregation of professionals and professional rivalry about supremacy of diagnosis is unhelpful to the debate and outmoded since it takes the search for the 'one cause' as its primary focus; the second is that understanding the problem of ADHD is entirely dependent on a multidisciplinary approach and on an active and continuing dialogue between professionals who are prepared to share their respective bodies of knowledge and understanding. Our workshops for parents, furthermore, have indicated that this group is often neglected as partners in the debate when in fact their participation is essential.

Once we enter into a discussion about a broader view of the behaviours associated with diagnosing ADHD, we lead towards a recognition of the importance of prevention. A focus on prevention and on understanding the physical, emotional, social and institutional factors that make children vulnerable is the cornerstone of this book.

We would like to emphasise that this book is not intended as the final and definitive word on the subject of ADHD. Instead we hope that it will provide the beginning of an ever-increasing dialogue and collaboration between professionals from different disciplines and points of view—as well as with parents—that does justice to the complexity of child development as well as child and family inter-action. The book takes as its starting point the consideration of different paradigms. This, we believe, is the fundamental prerequi-site for promoting child and family mental health and preventing childhood disorders in the twenty-first century.

How the book is organised

Chapter 2 introduces a neuropsychological approach to under-standing ADHD. By focusing on what we actually mean by attention, we help the reader to differentiate between what consti-tutes an attentional problem and what does not. We also focus on the difficulty of trying to achieve a differential diagnosis or to isolate a specific syndrome as opposed to understanding the complex needs of the child within a broader multidisciplinary context.

Chapter 3 presents a critique of the current conception of ADHD as a condition that can be completely described and treated under the medical model. Since medical diagnoses of ADHD represent the predominant mode of assessment and almost exclusively feature chemical treatment, we believe that it is timely to offer a critical assessment of this approach to the problem. In this chapter we also explore how the medicalisation of ADHD in many Western coun-tries might primarily reflect the growing cutbacks in health funding and other sociopolitical considerations.

Chapter 4 explores the risk factors for children within a social, organisational and cultural context and describes how these contribute to the expansion of ADHD as an illness of our time. It introduces the psychodynamic approach to understanding child development and the behavioural problems of children, including those commonly associated with ADHD.

Chapter 5 presents a framework based around the emotional milestones of development to describe how key attachment and relational processes are established between the parent and infant or young child. This chapter explores the impact of depression, loss, trauma and separation on these important developmental processes and explains how these experiences might create a 'rupture' for the child that has implications for the capacity for attention.

Chapter 6 explores the relevance of the concept of self-regulation as a more appropriate way of understanding some of the complex behaviours that are often diagnosed as ADHD—from a neuro-psychological view as well as from a psychodynamic perspective. Self-regulation is an important bridging concept, enabling us to create links between the development of brain function, particularly in infants and young children, and the way in which emotional experience is taken in and organised by the child. We refer to current research in this area, particularly on trauma and abuse, which throws light on the interplay between brain development and emotional experience.

Chapter 7 introduces a public health approach to understanding ADHD with a particular focus on the use of the biopsychosocial model. The primary advantage of such a model is that it is able to accept the heterogeneous nature of ADHD. This model moves us beyond the dichotomy of normal/pathological and acknowledges the need for multidisciplinary intervention. It features a proactive, preventive approach to problems of attention and impulse control using a community framework.

Chapter 8 poses the challenge of creating a fundamental paradigm shift in the delivery of services to children, parents and families in a new century. It considers the need for a different conceptual framework for understanding the nature of attentional problems in a changing society. In particular it emphasises the importance of including parents and children as stakeholders and full participants in finding solutions to their problems.

Chapter 9 presents practical recommendations for professionals working with children, parents and families, as well as for teachers in schools. These recommendations emphasise the importance of working in partnership with parents and the need for greater training in and understanding of child development for professionals in the field.

2

Neuropsychology and the diagnostic dilemmas of ADHD

The fundamental dilemma for paediatric neuropsychologists, as with nearly all of the medically oriented professionals who are called in to assist with the diagnosis of ADHD, is that there are no universally accepted biological markers for the condition. This would not be such a problem if there were a definitive *behavioural* test on which a diagnosis could be based, such as can be used, for example, in cases of suspected colour-blindness or hearing deficit. Unfortunately, despite the extensive training that neuropsychologists receive in psychometric test development and interpretation, no such definitive criterion test for ADHD currently exists, although there have been many attempts to isolate such a measure.

In the absence of a clearly defined biological marker, a gold standard neuropsychological test would need to be completely reliable (it would measure consistently on all occasions on which it is used) and completely valid (it would be able to distinguish clearly between those with the condition and those without). ADHD has been particularly resistant to reliable and valid diagnosis using neuropsychological tests, partly because of the fluctuating and multidimensional nature of the disorder's 'symptoms' (Barkley, 1998a) and partly because of continuing disagreement over the specific classificatory criteria for the condition (British Psychological Society, 1996).

First, the extent to which variable behaviour and performance is almost one of the defining characteristics of ADHD means that measures designed to produce a reliable score or rating are especially problematic with this group. While all human behaviour is variable and changes from day to day and across the contexts in which it is observed, it is usually still possible to draw conclusions about how an individual *typically* behaves, providing enough observations are taken. In fact the whole of the psychometric approach (that is, measuring mental states and processes) to assessment is based on this assumption. In the case of ADHD, behaviour and performance appear to either change excessively when there has been no change in the situation or stimuli, or else remain the same when circumstances or the demands of the task have changed (Barkley, 1998a). Normal approaches to psychological measurement that assume consistency of behaviour are unable to cope with this level of unreliability in the responses of the person being assessed.

Second, the extent to which disagreement continues over the fundamental nature of ADHD means that the validity of a diagnostic test can also be difficult to establish. No measure can be expected to perform accurately when the performance criteria are ambiguous or inconsistent. As will be demonstrated throughout this chapter, the definitional criteria for ADHD are still fuzzy and changeable, despite the passage of nearly one hundred years since the first scientific description of a group of children who appeared to demonstrate an 'abnormal incapacity for sustained attention, restlessness, fidgetiness, violent outbursts, destructiveness, non-compliance, choreiform movements, and minor congenital anomalies' (Still, 1902).

Notwithstanding the long history of scientific investigation of ADHD and its current position as the most commonly diagnosed psychiatric disorder in children, it is entirely understandable that significant debate still surrounds the diagnostic criteria for the condition. In ADHD we have a disorder that is defined by a number of heterogeneous, fluctuating and subjectively described behavioural characteristics that are unusually resistant to objective scientific measurement, yet apparently easily recognised and unusually disruptive within the general community. Given the ambiguous nature of the condition's symptoms and their proximity to deeply held notions of personal responsibility and self-control that exist in our community, it is little wonder that diagnostic decision making is encumbered with such a powerful political and emotional overlay, an overlay that has persisted ever since these children were first described by Still. In fact the validity of ADHD as an authentic psychiatric disorder is still questioned by many practitioners (see Armstrong, 1995; Kohn, 1989; Weinberg &

Brumback, 1992) and there is an ongoing sociological debate on the extent to which it represents a form of labelling designed to suppress nonconformity (Armstrong, 1993; Breggin, 1998). Much of this literature will be discussed in the following chapter, which presents a critique of the medical model as a useful framework for contemporary consideration of ADHD.

The diagnostic difficulties associated with the disorder are compounded by the expectations we hold for the clinical sciences. We live in an age when the same level of scientific measurement, explanation and control that appears to be available for events that occur in our physical world is demanded of troublesome psychological phenomena, despite the inherently complex and unpredictable nature of human behaviour. ADHD presents a unique challenge to psychologists because, while complete understanding of the disorder in a scientific sense demands a strict application of the reductionism on which the scientific method is based, the condition is one that at the present time is almost completely socially defined (Wakefield, 1992). While all science operates within a social framework, the complexity of the links between young people's attentional difficulties and the family, school and employment contexts in which they occur produces a tension that is not normally as obvious in other areas of scientific endeavour.

This chapter outlines some of the reasons for the continuing controversy surrounding the neuropsychological diagnosis of ADHD, and attempts to clarify some of the measurement issues that have dogged the field. We begin with a quick survey of the various diagnostic and explanatory approaches to the condition found in the contemporary literature.

The search for a biological marker

Although preoccupying the discipline since the condition was first identified by Still, the search for a clear *structural* difference in the brains of diagnosed children as a possible biological marker for ADHD has mostly been disappointing. Despite extensive contemporary research in this area, the one significant structural finding that has emerged so far has resulted from the use of magnetic resonance imaging (MRI). In this procedure the brain is exposed to a strong magnetic field that momentarily affects the spin of the hydrogen atoms in the water molecules within the brain cells. When the atoms return to their normal spin they release detectable signals that can be captured as computer-generated images. The result is a detailed picture of the brain's soft tissue.

These images have revealed that the normal 3 per cent advantage in volume of the right frontal lobe compared with the left is not present in many children who have been diagnosed with ADHD on behavioural criteria (Castellanos et al., 1994, 1996; Hynd et al., 1993). Occupying about one-third to one-fourth of the brain's mass, the frontal lobes are the largest of the brain structures in humans and the last to develop fully. The particular area of the frontal lobes that has been reported to be diminished in size in children with ADHD is the prefrontal cortex.

The prefrontal cortex, as the name suggests, is at the extreme anterior tip of the frontal lobes and is on the diagram on page 24. This area of the brain is the most recently evolved and has intricate and complex connections to all other areas of the brain and to all of the major sensory systems. It appears to be responsible for many of the higher cognitive functions such as language, planning, decision making and, most significantly, the self-monitoring of performance. Accumulating evidence suggests that the integrity of the prefrontal cortex is essential for the development of the verbal strategies that are used to guide and self-correct behaviour, direct and sustain attention, make complex judgements and inhibit impulsive responses to extraneous stimuli in the environment.

The finding by Castellanos and colleagues of reduced relative size in the right prefrontal cortex of children diagnosed with ADHD is significant because the functions associated with this structure are almost the exact deficits identified by Still at the beginning of the century. Unfortunately, in what will be seen as a consistent characteristic of reports such as these, the diagnostic utility of Castellanos' finding is limited by the fact that many children with ADHD do *not* exhibit reduced relative size in the prefrontal cortex. By the same token, there are many children who do not have the normal size differential reported by Castellanos but yet do not have ADHD. An additional reason to view these findings with some skepticism is that volumetric MRI is still at a fairly rudimentary stage of development and the reliability of the measurements that are produced by these procedures has been questioned by many researchers (Plante & Turkstra, 1991). Future research also needs to evaluate whether this measure is able to discriminate between children with ADHD and those with other common conditions such as conduct disorder and learning disability. None of the studies reported so far has included control groups of this nature and so the practical utility of the finding is limited.

With the increasing use of the newer radiological brain imaging techniques able to measure brain functioning, some differences have also been isolated among adults who were diagnosed with ADHD in childhood. *Functioning* in this sense refers to the actual neurological processes occurring within the central nervous system rather than to the neurological architecture of the brain itself. For example, in one of the most frequently cited studies in this field, Zametkin et al. (1990) used positron emission tomography (PET) to demonstrate that specific areas in the frontal lobes appear less active in these individuals than in 'normal' adults.

Although PET became available in the early 1980s, it remains primarily a research technique for constructing images of brain function by monitoring the movement and uptake of injected radioactive isotopes during various cognitive activities. The isotopes are attached to glucose molecules and their uptake in various parts of the brain paints a multicoloured 'picture' of cerebral functioning during various tasks. Two black and white images of PET scans are presented below.

Areas of white surrounded by dark fringes indicate high uptake of the glucose molecules, and therefore high activity. The second image is of the brain of an adult with 'residual' ADHD, observed from above during a simple planning task. The first image is of a normal control during the same task. Notice the higher levels of frontal lobe activity in the normal control.

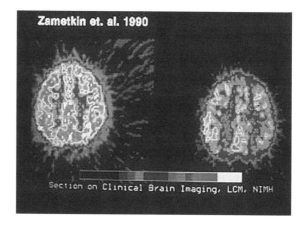

Zametkin et. al. 1990

Section on Clinical Brain Imaging, LCM, NIMH

Despite the publicity that Zametkin's finding received, its practical utility is limited because the dangers associated with radioactive substances mean that the procedure cannot be routinely used with children. A more serious difficulty is the strong likelihood that adults with residual ADHD represent a subgroup who may well have had a more severe or unusual variety of the paediatric condition. In fact an attempt to replicate this research with adolescents has not been successful (Zametkin et al., 1993) and other research has suggested that the original findings might have been an artifact owing to gender differences in the sample. The control group for this study consisted mainly of females.

There are other measures of brain functioning sometimes employed by clinicians to assist in diagnosis of ADHD, although similar problems have been encountered with these procedures. Electroencephalographs (EEGs), for example, are used to detect electrical activity in different parts of the brain. One EEG technique involves presenting the child with a visual or auditory stimulus and determining the appropriateness of the brain waves (commonly referred to as evoked potentials) emitted through the scalp. Research suggests that many children with ADHD demonstrate decreased amplitudes in the micro-voltages of these evoked potentials, faster habituation to the stimulus and increased slow wave activity (Klorman, 1991; Lahat et al., 1995). In addition to this general 'sluggishness' in brain activity, these children appear to demonstrate slower (and more variable) reaction times to both visual and auditory stimuli.

While these results present a uniform picture of lower levels of cerebral arousal in those affected by the condition, it is also the case that many non-ADHD children exhibit similar abnormalities in EEG activity and in reaction times when undergoing the same diagnostic procedures. This lack of specificity in the available measures haunts the entire field of ADHD research and is a major source of frustration for clinicians as well as for investigators hoping to isolate a single, clear biological marker for the condition that may be used in diagnosis. *Specificity* in a diagnostic sense refers to the capacity of a clinical measure to discriminate between those who have the disorder and those who don't, while *sensitivity* merely refers to the measure's ability to identify those who have the disorder. Often these two characteristics are in dynamic tension with each other because the more sensitive measures are also more likely to mis-classify normal children and vice versa. In fact many of the common procedures used to diagnose ADHD lack both sensitivity and specificity, despite the claims many clinicians make for the diagnostic information they provide.

The frequent observation that, as a group, children with ADHD suffer higher incidences of disorders such as incontinence, somatic complaints, allergies, colds, urinary tract infections and sleep disturbances is also useful knowledge for clinicians and perhaps hints at the condition's biological origins (Cantwell & Hanna, 1989). Once again, however, the actual diagnostic utility of this information is compromised for the same reasons that brain imaging, EEG, or reaction time measures have been found to be problematic. That is, while these problems frequently coexist with ADHD, they cannot be used to pinpoint the presence of the condition in any one child and they appear to be more common in nearly all groups of psychiatrically ill children.

Most of the evidence suggesting a biological cause of ADHD is derived from the common observation that over 75 per cent of diagnosed children appear to respond positively to stimulant therapy with dexamphetamine or methylphenidate hydrochloride (Green, Wong & Atkins, 1999). In fact it is this finding that has led many medical practitioners to view stimulant therapy as a valid diagnostic challenge with children. That is, the treatment itself has become the diagnostic tool so that those who do respond are presumed to have the condition and vice versa.

The supposed high rate of positive response to stimulants has also prompted a number of theories suggesting that important neurotransmitters are either depleted or dysfunctional in those with ADHD. Neurotransmitters are the naturally produced chemical substances that allow electrical impulses to travel across the synapse from one nerve cell in the brain to another. Neurotransmitter disturbances could theoretically produce many of the cognitive difficulties experienced by those with the condition and explain the positive results produced by the stimulants.

Generally speaking, dopamine is the neurotransmitter targeted by the most commonly used stimulants although the medications differ in how they increase dopamine concentrations in the synapse. Dexamphetamine appears to release newly synthesised dopamine and to block its re-uptake, while methylphenidate releases stored dopamine (Shenker, 1992). This differential effect may partly explain why some children appear to respond to one of the drugs and not to the other, although most studies report that both treatments produce similar overall results (Shukla & Otten, 1999).

The theories proposing that the dopamine neurotransmitters are either depleted or dysfunctional in those with ADHD are vulnerable on a number of counts. First, urine analyses conducted on those diagnosed with ADHD have found no differences in the amount of excreted metabolites (by-products) of these neurotransmitters in these children compared with others (Baker et al., 1993). Second, the evidence suggesting a high rate of positive response to stimulant therapy tends to be derived from studies conducted with methodologies in which there has been no attempt to 'blind' patients, parents or therapists to the treatment being offered. This allows the possibility that an unknown component of the therapeutic benefit from these pharmacological interventions is derived from a strong placebo effect. Such placebo effects in the drug treatment of ADHD are reported to average about 20 per cent (Ullman & Sleator, 1986) although there are some reports of up to a 40 per cent rate of positive response to dummy pills.

An additional point is that, while the calming effect of stimulant therapy was once believed to be a unique and paradoxical response of children with ADHD, it is now clear that nearly all children and adults register increased attentional capacity after taking either of the two commonly prescribed stimulants (Peloquin & Klorman, 1986; Rapoport et al., 1978; Yelich & Salamone, 1994). Therefore it is doubtful whether responsiveness to stimulants in and of itself provides enough evidence to assist diagnosis or to suggest that the condition is unambiguously caused by a deficit in those substances. Even the American National Institute of Health consensus statement (NIH, 1998), which takes an unambiguously 'medical' view of the condition, cautioned against the diagnostic use of stimulants with the statement that 'some practitioners invalidly use response to medication as a diagnostic criterion'.

Qualitative observations, behavioural ratings and psychometric tests

With the current absence of any reliable physical or biological markers to indicate pathology, practitioners are reduced to a dependence on qualitative observations, behavioural ratings and psychometric tests. The benefits and disadvantages of each of these diagnostic approaches to ADHD will be considered in the next section.

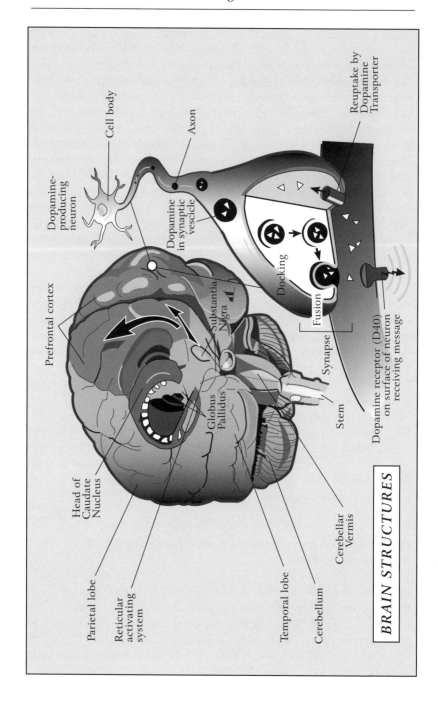

BRAIN STRUCTURES

Qualitative observations

The observational criteria that comprise the most frequently utilised diagnostic framework—the *Diagnostic and Statistical Manual*, 4th Edition (DSM-IV) (American Psychiatric Association, 1994)—seem to be clearly presented, and on the surface it is a very straight-forward process to find the necessary behaviours that qualify a child for the ADHD label. The criteria are reproduced in Appendix 1 of this book, and it can be seen that these behaviours typically fall under the general categories of: a) inattention or inconsistent atten-tion and b) hyperactivity–impulsivity.

Unfortunately, as was suggested in the introduction to this chapter, these observational criteria as represented in DSM-IV appear to be almost as unreliable as the biological markers for which they are substitutes. This unreliability is indicated in practical terms by the extreme variability that exists in the rates of diagnosis produced by physicians within the same locality as well as across state and national boundaries. Examples of this variability were presented in Chapter 1 and, rather than reflecting a genuine vari-ability in the incidence of the condition, they more likely represent substantial differences in the way observational criteria are being interpreted.

Some of the cross-national variance in rates of diagnosis can be accounted for by the use of different criteria for the condition. Most workers in European settings use the diagnostic systems of the World Health Organization *International Classification of Diseases*, 10th Edition (ICD-10) (WHO, 1993). Under this taxonomy the equiv-alent category to ADHD is hyperkinetic disorder, a term that relates directly back to the original focus on disordered control of movement described by Still (1902). The ICD criteria for hyper-kinetic disorder are presented in Appendix 2 of this book and it can be seen that one reason for the lower percentage of 'cases' in European settings might be the exclusion from the diagnostic net of those exhibiting comorbidity. That is, the ICD criteria specifically exclude children whose attentional problems are associated with conduct, mood, anxiety or pervasive developmental disorder. It is important to recognise, however, that trans-Atlantic inconsistencies in rates of ADHD diagnosis remain even when the same criteria are used by clinicians from European and American settings. For example, Prendergast et al. (1988) compared rates of ADHD diag-nosis in British and American practitioners using the same criteria and found that a similar differential prevailed, with American clinicians apparently more willing to recognise the symptoms in their patients.

Inconsistencies in rates of ADHD diagnosis deserve considerable attention because they go to the heart of the controversies that have surrounded the condition over the past two decades. Some explanations have focused on the extent to which strict diagnostic criteria are actually followed by clinicians. For example, Wolraich et al. (1990) argue that less than half of all physicians in the USA actually use the DSM criteria as the basis for their ADHD decision making so that diagnostic consistency is not even to be expected. Similar inconsistency in the employment of diagnostic procedures can be expected in other countries and so idiosyncratic use of measures might be a major factor in producing some of the apparent geographical variability of the condition.

The diversity in the actual DSM observational criteria for diagnosis of ADHD provides another possible reason for the inconsistency. While these criteria have undergone continuous refinement since they were first published in 1980, with the current requirement that any six of the nine inattention and any six of the nine hyperactivity–impulsivity criteria be met, a very large number of behavioural permutations in the condition are possible, so that consistency would be hard to recognise, even if it was present. A dozen children could present with a wide diversity of 'symptoms' and yet receive the same diagnosis so that the existence of a reliable underlying ADHD syndrome might often not appear immediately obvious to those who observe the results of diagnostic decision making.

Lack of precision in the language used to describe the diagnostic requirements for ADHD in each of the taxonomies is also a possible source of inconsistency. Both the ICD and DSM diagnostic systems rely on practitioners to interpret the term 'often' in relation to the target behaviours for ADHD. For example, the requirement that the child 'often appears not to listen to what is being said' is an item appearing in both sets of criteria. Yet there are no guidelines presented as to the actual number that 'often' in this context represents. It is left up to the clinical judgement of the practitioner to determine what 'often' refers to in the context of the child's level of development, yet we know from many years of research that individual perceptions can vary dramatically, even among highly trained and experienced professionals. While one paediatrician might believe that three instances of not listening in a day constitutes 'often' for a seven-year-old, another might believe that six such occurrences are not unusual. Equally as important is the issue of how 'not listening' is to be objectively defined. No specifications for this behaviour are provided and the other symptoms described in the ADHD criteria such as fidgeting, distractibility and forgetfulness are equally open to extreme variability in interpretation.

The way in which the diagnostician gathers information about the ADHD criterion behaviours from parents and teachers is another obvious source of inconsistency. Unstructured clinical interviews with parents and children are notoriously unreliable with respect to diagnostic decision making (Hinshaw, 1994). Individual differences in interviewer orientation and style combine with the inevitable fluctuations that occur in respondent mood and perspective to ensure unacceptable variability in the characteristics of children receiving the ADHD label after the application of this diagnostic process.

Even structured interviews in which the diagnostician systematically presents the respondent with questions stemming directly from the specified DSM criteria arranged in a consistent order have their limitations in terms of reliability and validity. They often focus exclusively on parental concerns and behavioural reports to the neglect of information from other settings and sometimes the subjectivity of these parental accounts is difficult to reference to a 'normal' baseline. Specific problems with the reliability and validity of information collected from a single source are outlined below.

Rating scales

Standardised rating scales attempt to remedy many of these deficiencies in the collection of behavioural data and they have become the fastest growing assessment tool in developmental psychology (Kamphaus, Petoskey & Rowe, 2000). While both the ICD and the DSM diagnostic systems are by definition categorical in their approach to ADHD (that is, the child either has the condition or doesn't, depending on whether the criteria are met), many neuropsychologists prefer to conceptualise the disorder as existing on a continuum. With this approach, each of the diagnostically significant behaviours are quantified by raters using some meaningful scale (such as never–0, sometimes 1–2, often 3–5) and the ratings are totalled for each dimension being measured. These totals are referenced to a normal distribution within each age-level so that cut-off points can be applied and the decision about the unusualness of the behaviour made on a statistical basis. Unfortunately, while such approaches are meant to improve the consistency and reliability of ADHD diagnosis, it appears that rating scales are susceptible to many of the same problems that have been documented for the diagnostic systems discussed above.

Data collected on rating scales can be judged on two criteria, interobserver reliability and interobserver agreement. While these attributes are similar, they actually refer to two different indices of consistency and each needs to be discussed separately in relation to the ADHD scales often used with children. Interobserver reliability simply refers to the degree to which raters vary together in their estimate of a particular behaviour. If two observers are rating the frequency of ADHD symptoms on a scale and one always underestimates while the other consistently overestimates, the scale would still appear to be reliable because the ratings would move in the same direction for each item. While it might seem misleading and overly generous to use this as an index of a measure's consistency, reviews of commonly used children's rating scales suggest that even on this relatively lenient criterion, the correlation between raters is typically only about .4. This coefficient can be interpreted to mean that a maximum of 16 per cent of the judgements made by one person about a child covary with the judgements of another about the same child. The percentage of shared variability declines even further if the respondents come from different settings, for example family and school (Achenbach, McConaughy & Howell, 1987).

In contrast to interobserver reliability, interobserver agreement refers to the extent to which each observer nominates the same score for each behaviour. So, in the case of the item 'How often does this child appear not to listen to what is being said?' interobserver agreement would only occur if both raters chose the *same* frequency category in their response to the scale. Not surprisingly this much stricter definition of consistency is often neglected in reports of the reliability of ADHD rating scales and indices of interobserver agreement on target behaviours are notoriously low (Barkley, 1990).

An index of interobserver agreement has the advantage of taking into account the bias as well as the inconsistency in the way the observers use the scale. While inconsistency is often referred to as *random* measurement error, bias is a more *systematic* source of error and, in the context of psychopathology, such systematic error occurs at the intersection between the condition and its social context. Many examples of bias in the assessment of ADHD have been documented.

For example, Stevens (1981) found systematic variability in the 'hyperactivity' ratings collected from trained psychologists who had all viewed the same film depicting a boy's behaviour within a school setting but had read different biographical histories of the child. In each of these fictitious biographies his socioeconomic status had been systematically manipulated. The psychologists consistently rated the behaviour of the boy when he was labelled lower-class as more hyperactive than when he was described as a middle- and upper-class boy.

The bias described above is an example of the 'halo/horns' effect, a common source of psychometric error where characteristics other than those specifically being measured influence the ratings provided by practitioners, parents and teachers. The 'horns effect' appears to be a particular problem with scales designed to assist in ADHD diagnosis because children presenting with almost *any* disruptive behaviour tend to be rated higher on 'attentional problems' by teachers, even when the problematic behaviours are unrelated to inattentiveness or overactivity (Abikoff, Courtney, Pelham & Koplewicz, 1994; Schachar, Sandberg & Rutter, 1986). As a general rule, rating scales tend to overestimate the prevalence of attentional dysfunction in the community because the existence of almost any behavioural problem in a child results in exaggerated ratings of inattention or hyperactivity.

The variability in rating scale scores commonly found with ADHD might also reflect systematic variability in the tolerance levels of the observers making the ratings, even when the supposedly 'objective' DSM criteria are met. For example, a child demonstrating 'forgetfulness' or 'disorganisation' is less likely to be noticed within the family than in a school setting where learning and the development of self-responsibility often carries a higher priority. There have been extensive reports of such inconsistency between ADHD ratings collected from educational and family settings (Lahey, McBurnett & Piacentini, 1987) and even within schools there is variability across teachers and across departments. It is known, for example, that special education teachers are more tolerant of disruptive behaviours in children than are generalist teachers and so they are likely to rate the severity of such behaviours lower on rating scales (Safran & Safran, 1987).

Similar variability in levels of tolerance for disruption operate within and across families. Evidence suggests that mothers are more likely to report symptoms of ADHD in their children than are fathers;

that identical behaviours are less likely to be reported as symptoms in the morning than in the afternoon; and that older parents have a lower threshold for reporting behavioural deviance than their younger peers (Barkley, 1997a). Even the children themselves are biased in their self ratings, possibly because difficulty in self-monitoring one's own behaviour is one of the commonly reported characteristics of the condition. For example, Loeber, Green, Lahey and Strouthamer-Loeber (1991) report that children with difficulties related to attention and hyperactivity consistently understate the frequency of their ADHD symptoms relative to mainstream children.

There are also dramatic cross-cultural differences in perceptions of inappropriate behaviour. When standardised videotape vignettes of children participating in individual and group activities were rated by clinicians from a variety of cultural backgrounds, Mann et al. (1992) reported that Chinese and Indonesian clinicians gave consistently higher hyperactivity ratings than did their Japanese and American colleagues. These findings suggest that the thresholds for deviance, among both clinicians and informants responding to well standard-ised ADHD scales, have strong cultural determinants that could have a bearing on the international differences in rates of diagnosis.

An additional source of diagnostic unreliability, touched on earlier, stems from the nature of the condition itself because children with ADHD tend to demonstrate unusual levels of fluctuation in their behaviour and performance (Douglas, 1972; 1983). This increased variability has been noted across settings as well as across time periods within the same setting, and fluctuating performance has even been suggested as a primary marker for the condition (Barkley, 1990). In addition to creating a further source of frustration for parents and teachers ('He was able to do this yesterday!'), the 'reliable unreliability' that characterises the behaviour of these children acts to confound conventional diagnostic procedures based on observational criteria. Even those test and observational techniques with well established high standards of psychometric reliability have trouble measuring the behaviour of 'unreliable' examinees.

In spite of these problems, rating scales filled out by parents or teachers are probably the most common source of information used by practitioners making diagnostic decisions. Many clinicians simply use an informal scale abbreviated from the DSM-IV criteria while others adopt more formal instruments. Examples of the more commonly used behaviour rating scales include the *Child Behaviour Checklist* (Achenbach, 1991), the *Conners' Rating Scales—Revised*

(Conners, 1997) and the *Behavioural Rating Inventory* (Rowe & Rowe, 1995). The reliability of many of these measures has been questioned in the literature, although it must be remembered that whatever scale is used, the nature of the condition means that ratings of children's behaviour should be obtained from as many different informants as possible. The reliability of all measures increases in direct proportion to the number and variety of observations that are taken and often the contrast between the parent and teacher ratings of the same child can be valuable diagnostic information in itself. For example, higher teacher reports of disturbance compared with parent ratings might indicate that the child behaves adequately in the more individualised one-to-one home environment while becoming disorganised and hyperactive in the more ambiguous and non-responsive school setting.

The international, interstate, inter-clinician and inter-informant differences in diagnostic tendencies when the decision is based on rating scale scores might partly reflect the fact that the behavioural manifestations of ADHD cannot be simply dichotomised into what is normal and what is pathological—especially when considered within a developmental and social context. Psychologists, perhaps more so than medically oriented clinicians, tend to favour the view that the behaviours that are supposed to characterise the condition, along with most aspects of human functioning, can only be placed along a continuum where opinion regarding their pathology fluctuates over situations, the age of the child and time at which the behaviour is observed. Behaviour that at one time or place would be considered maladaptive might, in the case of another child or in different circumstances or culture, be considered perfectly normal. For example, it has been claimed that, 'at some ages, 50% or more of normal children are perceived by adults as showing various signs of hyperactivity' (Whalen & Henker, 1996).

These findings have prompted many workers in the field to move away from any attempt to isolate ADHD in a particular child using a simple rating scale. Instead they adopt an approach to diagnosing the condition that relies upon the observance of 'misfit' between the temperament of the child and that of the parent or teacher. These 'ecological' or 'transactional' assessment models rely heavily on the investigations of Chess and Thomas (1989) regarding the early appearance of temperament in children. According to this research all humans exhibit a set of temperament traits that are largely present from birth in attributes such as activity level, adaptability and regularity; tendency to approach or withdraw in novel situations; intensity of reactions and mood; persistence and attention span, distractibility and sensory threshold. All traits vary normally in the general population; however, certain temperaments are particularly likely to induce a 'poor fit' with the values and expectations of caretakers. Children with this 'difficult' temperament cluster (low adaptability and regularity, negative mood, high intensity, etc.) are more likely to develop social problems and transactional stress, but this might only happen in situations of extreme misfit. It is these 'misfitting' children who tend to receive the diagnosis of ADHD.

Psychometric tests

In a different approach to dealing with the unreliability that characterises the condition and its measurement, attempts have been made to standardise the situational variables that appear to influence the occurrence of ADHD symptoms by using formal one-to-one psychometric testing. The advantage of this testing is that it takes a sample of a child's behaviour in a rigidly controlled environment so that performance can be 'objectively' measured and related directly to the attentional disturbances that are presumed to lie at the heart of the condition. With the use of standardised tests, a decision about abnormality can then be made on a statistical basis, recognising that cognitive attributes, along with the behaviours that are measured with rating scales, tend to exhibit a characteristic bell-shaped normal distribution rather than clustering in those who have been diagnosed. Aberrance is simply the lowest tip of the distributional performance curve.

Of course the disadvantage of a psychometric testing approach is that gains in reliability are often achieved at a cost to validity. Just as the standardised observations made of a child's behaviour in the clinician's rooms are unlikely to reflect the 'real-world' behaviour of the child, so too the results of one-to-one psychometric testing provide only an approximation of the child's level of performance on 'real-world' tasks. Neuropsychological testing is therefore often criticised for its lack of 'ecological validity' (Barkley, 1992) in the sense that the generalisability of the 'score' is often heavily compromised.

In spite of these problems with generalisability, neuropsychological testing of the child's capacity to utilise their attentional resources can be a valuable component of the diagnostic process, provided the test results are structured in some way that accords with our knowledge of how the brain processes information. This is especially so because empirical research, using both animal and human models, has increasingly supported the view that attention is not a single construct but an ability that can be divided into a number of linked components. While there are many models that integrate the components of attention in different ways (Barkley, 1996; Cooley & Morris, 1990; Douglas, 1983; Halperin, 1996; Posner, 1988; Sergeant, 1996; Shiffrin & Schneider, 1977; van Zomeren & Brouwer, 1994), the so-called 'Mirsky model' is gaining increasing recognition as an especially useful perspective from which to examine attention in both adults and children. The utility of such a model derives from its capacity to provide a way of thinking about ADHD that encourages a systematic analysis of the diverse clinical symptoms that comprise the syndrome, instead of viewing the condition as the result of a single biological deficit. Such an approach means that there is less chance of the clinician relying solely on biomedical treatment and a greater likelihood that the specific deficits will be addressed in a manner that is more appropriate to the nature of the presenting problems and their likely diverse aetiology.

The Mirsky model of attention

The 'Mirsky model' has been extensively studied (Mirsky, 1996; Mirsky, Anthony, Duncan, Ahearn & Kellam, 1991) and is based upon the factor analytic results of research carried out with a standard battery of multiple, well normed neuropsychological measures. Factor analysis is a statistical procedure that determines the degree of correlation between performances on various tasks to determine the extent to which they reflect particular underlying characteristics, known as 'factors'. The results of these investigations are summarised below, together with references to the measures used to identify each component and tentative suggestions of where these functions might be localised in the brain. The four elements extracted by the Mirsky model were (a) sustain (b) focus execute (c) shift (d) encode.

Sustained attention

The capacity to maintain focus and alertness over time is referred to as sustained attention, an ability that normally matures relatively early in children. This aspect of attention is often conceptualised as 'vigilance' and there is much evidence to suggest that children with attention disorders experience particular difficulty with this skill, resulting in what is often called a 'short attention span' (Barkley 1992).

Sustained attention is most commonly measured on computerised tasks in which the child is asked to monitor a video screen for prolonged periods and to respond to the appearance of randomly presented visual or auditory stimuli by pressing appropriate switches. This sort of task is often referred to as a *Continuous Performance Test* or CPT, and children with ADHD tend, as the test progresses, to make more omission and commission errors than other children. In other words the rate at which their scores deteriorate with time spent on the task declines faster than appears to be the case with normal children at a similar level of development.

There are a number of continuous performance tests commercially available, including the *Conners' Continuous Performance Test* (Conners, 1995), the *TOVA* (Test of Variables of Attention—Greenberg & Waldman, 1993), and the *Vigil Continuous Performance Test* (Psychological Corporation, 1996). In fact the main difficulty with these tests from a diagnostic point of view is the variety of versions adopted among practitioners and researchers, which leads to a confusing range of numbers used to describe a child's performance. On some of the measures there is also a problem with the inadequate standardisation employed in the test development process (Riccio, Reynolds & Lowe, 2001).

It is believed that the capacity for sustained attention is associated with an optimal level of cortical arousal. This capacity is the major responsibility of the reticular activating system (RAS), which is composed of nuclei and fibres that pass through the brainstem, diencephalon and the frontal cortex. While certainly not a significant source of candidates for the diagnostic label of ADHD, damage to the RAS, particularly during the prenatal period, has been associated with later attentional problems (Douglas, 1983; Zentall, 1975). Other midbrain structures involved in maintaining attention are the thalamus and the limbic system, particularly the hippocampus (Thompson & Bettinger, 1970).

Selective or focused attention

The ability to focus on a specific target for enhanced processing so that the resulting information can be responded to appropriately is referred to as 'selective' or 'focused' attention. Often children suffering from attentional difficulties might be able to demonstrate this capacity until competing information becomes present. It is in this situation that the 'filtering' element might begin to break down and the child feels bombarded by environmental stimulation with no capacity to find structure or meaning. This function is commonly tested by neuropsychologists using tasks in which the target stimuli are embedded in an array of conflicting and inappropriate response stimuli. The *Letter Cancellation Test* (LCT) is one such task. This is a simple paper and pencil test that requires the child to mark a specific pair of letters that are repeatedly presented within a random array of other letters. The capacity to perform adequately on these sorts of tasks appears to be partly determined by the integrity of the temporal and parietal areas of the brain (shown in the diagram on page 22).

Shifting attention

The ability to change attentive focus in a flexible and adaptive manner is commonly referred to as shifting attention, although some of the neuropsychological literature describes the inability to effectively supervise attentional control as a deficit in the executive functions or the central executive. There is considerable debate about whether this aspect of attention is deficient in children with ADHD, possibly because it is considered to be a comparatively late developing ability and the DSM criteria specify that the condition needs to be apparent early in the child's life (before age seven). The view that ADHD primarily represents an executive function deficit has been taken up recently by a number of high profile researchers in the field and so some of this evidence will be reviewed in more depth in Chapter 6, especially as the executive functions are generally considered to involve other skills beyond the capacity to shift attention. It is interesting to note that these same researchers have recommended that the maximum age hurdle necessary for consideration of an ADHD diagnosis be raised from seven to thirteen in the next revision of the DSM criteria (Barkley, 1997a).

Shifting attention is mostly measured on tasks that require the child to move frequently from one category of response to another. These tasks usually involve some element of sorting, where responses have to vary according to criteria that are constantly changing. Commonly used instruments include the *Wisconsin Card Sorting Test* (WCST: Heaton, 1981), where the rule for sorting cards changes without warning from being based on colours, to shapes and finally to numbers, the *Go, No-Go* test where criteria for action shift on a moment-by-moment basis, and the *Contingency Naming Test* (CNT: Taylor, 1988), a relatively new test that involves holding two opposing rules in mind and acting on one rule in some circumstances and the opposite way in others. On each of these tests either the number of errors or the length of time taken to complete the full test is frequently accepted as a measure of the ability to shift attention, an ability that is usually localised in the prefrontal areas of the brain.

Speed of encoding and information processing

The rate at which information from the environment is registered and then outputted via motor activities is referred to as the speed of information processing. As indicated earlier in this chapter, some children diagnosed with ADHD are found to be sluggish in their response times to auditory and visual stimuli, while others are merely erratic. Many are both slow and irregular. Response times are typically measured on the same computerised CPT tasks used to gauge the capacity of the child to sustain attention but a different measure is used to index the stability or reliability of the attentional system. This capacity has been tentatively located by Mirsky et al. in the midline thalamic structures and in the brainstem.

With the increasing recognition of the importance of these components of attention, a number of omnibus tests that provide standardised scores for children on these attributes are in the process of development. One such measure is the *Test of Everyday Attention in Children* (TEACh), a well normed instrument that examines all of the elements of attention described above. This test is a downward extension of a similar test used with adults and represents a significant attempt to tease out some of the complexity from the attention construct. Research has indicated that this measure is capable of identifying children who have been previously diagnosed with ADHD by clinicians (Manly et al., 1999).

General tests of cognitive ability

In addition to these specialised instruments, neuropsychologists typically utilise standardised tests of general ability such as the *Wechsler Intelligence Scale for Children* (WISC). As well as providing an indication of the extent to which a child's attentional problems are related to overall cognitive capacity, these measures have two subtests on which adequate performance is presumed to be at least partly determined by the ability of the child to resist distraction. The latest revision of the scale (the WISC III) combines the scores on these two subtests into what has become known as the *Freedom from Distraction Index* (Wechsler, 1991), an index that is frequently used to assist in ADHD diagnosis. While this index has been shown to be sensitive to ADHD (Prifitera & Dersh, 1993), an unfortunate problem is that it appears to be just as sensitive to learning disability. This means that it is not useful for discriminating children with learning disorders from children with attentional disorders (Wielkiewicz, 1990) and so cannot be used in any definitive sense for diagnosing the condition.

The difficulties associated with the use of formal psychometric tests to diagnose a condition in which a primary characteristic is the tendency for performance levels to fluctuate excessively have already been mentioned. As this intraindividual performance variability occurs across both time and setting, a child's test score might appear normal or abnormal, depending on when and where he or she was tested. These difficulties are further compounded by the tendency for a formal test to artificially curb the expression of this performance variability through the moderating presence of the test administrator. Most of the problems experienced by children with ADHD occur in ambiguous and unstructured situations whereas a psychometric test by its very nature is a structured situation in which the child is directed to perform a series of tasks in a set sequence by an adult. Thus the formality of the test situation and the presence of the clinician can compensate for the attentional problems of the child, attenuating an important piece of diagnostic information. On the previously described Continuous Performance Test, for example, scores are known to differ dramatically according to whether or not the examiner is present during assessment (Draeger, Prior & Sanson, 1986; Power, 1992) and so during formal psychometric testing the clinician is said to be acting as a de facto set of frontal lobes for the child in helping them keep on task.

Specific measures of impulsivity/hyperactivity

While predominantly employed for research purposes, activity and seat movement recorders are sometimes used to assess levels of overall activity in children and these devices have been found to be useful in distinguishing ADHD from other child psychiatric disorders (Halperin et al., 1992). They are electronic devices that are worn by the child for set periods of time so that objective information about activity levels can be compared with normative data. More sophisticated devices that operate on the same principle monitor head movements while the child is performing the Continuous Performance Test. These instruments are also sometimes used to evaluate the impact of interventions and they are capable of recording fairly subtle changes in a child's behaviour after the administration of psychostimulants.

Although pedometers and head movement monitors represent an attempt to measure the hyperactivity component of ADHD electronically, the most commonly used 'paper and pencil' measure of impulsivity is the *Matching Familiar Figures Test* (MFFT: Kagan, 1966). The MFFT is a twelve-item measure of impulse control, visual discrimination and attention to detail. The child is shown a picture of an object and must choose from a group of nearly identical pictures the one that exactly matches the target picture. Scoring is based on the speed of response in relation to accuracy. Children with ADHD are reported to respond quickly to each item while at the same time making many errors, which results in an overall low score (Sonuga-Barke, Houlberg & Hall, 1994). Impulsivity is also sometimes measured on the Continuous Performance Test where premature responses to stimuli (children responding before the signals actually appear on the screen) are monitored.

Attempts to measure impulsivity most clearly demonstrate the ambiguous nature of ADHD symptomatology because impulsivity is a notoriously difficult concept to pin down in a measurement sense. While it is clear that there is a developmental aspect to the capacity of individuals to inhibit initial impulses and to cognitively reflect before committing to action, impulsivity can also be seen as a positive capacity to respond quickly to environmental demands and feedback. In many cases, too much reflection before initiating adaptive action might be seen as dysfunctional 'rigidity' or as a pathological symptom of emotional disorders. These problematic aspects find expression in the difficulties that have been encountered using the MFFT. Despite being used in over 800 studies of impulsivity, this test has received extensive psychometric criticism for its inability to reliably identify pathology, for its high correlation with intelligence and for its poor reliability. Other scales that have been devised to measure impulsivity have been forced to discriminate between *functional* and *dysfunctional* impulsivity, in an acknowledgement that acting before thinking can be advantageous in some circumstances (Dickman, 1993).

Other diagnostic issues

Perhaps the greatest dilemma facing developmental neuropsychologists working in the field of ADHD is the fact that individuals receiving the same diagnosis do not appear to represent a homogeneous group. Even after allowing for variable interpretations of the diagnostic criteria across settings and observers, the condition appears to be typically confounded with a variety of other developmental disorders. Over a quarter of all children diagnosed with ADHD have a concurrent diagnosis of learning disability, and 'attentional difficulties' are frequently experienced by children with other conditions such as autism, Tourette's syndrome and mental retardation (Shaywitz & Shaywitz, 1991; Weinberg & Emslie, 1991). In fact it is the extent of this association of ADHD with other developmental disorders that accounts for much of the variability in incidence rates across settings and cultures commented upon earlier in this chapter.

We also know that children with a variety of *physical* disorders tend also to experience attention problems. Head injury, encephalitis, meningitis, epilepsy, phenylketonuria (PKU—a congenital metabolic disease) and diabetes have all been associated with deficits in this aspect of information processing. In addition, there are a number of treatments for relatively common medical conditions that result in attentional problems for many children. Examples of such treatments are the irradiation of the brain that some children receive for acute lymphoblastic leukaemia, surgery in which parts of the brain are excised and several drug regimens.

Emotional disorders are also frequently confounded with attentional difficulties. Some studies have reported that up to 60 per cent of children with ADHD present with diagnosable oppositional/defiant behaviour, a fact reflected in the greater tendency of European clinicians, relative to their American counterparts, to diagnose conduct disorder in preference to ADHD. American reviews of the literature have concluded that oppositional/defiant or conduct disorders coexist with ADHD in approximately 35 per cent of children

(Green, Wong & Atkins, 1999), while a study conducted by Anderson et al. (1987) in New Zealand found that 47 per cent of children with ADHD had these difficulties as co-occurring diagnoses.

Anxiety and depression are also prevalent disorders comorbid with the condition. The same American review cited above estimated that approximately 25 per cent of children diagnosed with ADHD had a coexisting anxiety disorder and that 18 per cent were depressed (Green, Wong & Atkins, 1999). The New Zealand study conducted by Anderson et al. found 26 per cent of ADHD children with these disorders.

The extent of the comorbidity of other conditions with ADHD, together with the degree to which *attention* is affected by the myriad of medical and psychiatric disturbances to which children are prone, underlines the difficulties associated with attempts to reliably diagnose the disorder. Attention is an incredibly complex cognitive function that has been the focus of literally thousands of articles and books since the birth of psychology as a formal science in the latter half of the nineteenth century. One of the reasons that attention has been so intensively studied for such a long period of time is that problems with focusing, maintaining or shifting attention have so great an impact on our everyday lives. It is only to be expected that a deficit in a cognitive function, upon which we rely so much, should attract the interest of those looking to explain the wide diversity of cognitive, emotional and behavioural disturbances to which children are susceptible.

While the construct of attention has acted as a lightning rod for reports of childhood disability in a multitude of different forms, we have tried to demonstrate that the measurement issues associated with this aspect of performance have cast doubt on its specific utility in ADHD diagnostic decision making. To state that these children suffer from a deficit in attention does not really clarify the exact nature of their disability and a sophisticated approach to assessment is demanded for the term to have any meaning at all.

The extent of the influence that physical and social surroundings have on levels of attention also means that problems in this area of functioning cannot be looked at in isolation. Approaches to the assessment and diagnosis of attentional problems that do not take into account their wider social and family context are bound to reveal only half of the ADHD story. In the next chapter we present a critique of the medical model, an exceptionally limited approach to ADHD that attempts to do just this.

3

A critique of the medical model

The medical model is a particular way of thinking about disturbances in physical and mental functioning that accepts the utility of the disease analogy. Approaches originating from this perspective concentrate exclusively on the diagnosis and treatment of the underlying biological processes that are believed to result in the appearance of the pathological 'symptoms', which become the focus of the clinician's attention. The medical model takes an exclusively individual perspective and emphasises the application of technology and pharmacology to disease.

While the medical model has been undeniably successful in a scientific sense over the two hundred or so years in which it has prevailed in Western culture, the continuing utility of this reductionistic approach is beginning to be questioned. In the case of physical illness, rapidly expanding knowledge of the behavioural and social factors that are associated with the occurrence of many bodily disturbances has prompted a reappraisal of the dominance of the medical perspective.

One aspect of this reappraisal concerns the false credit the medical model has taken for the dramatic improvement that has occurred in the physical health of populations. In fact the longer life spans we now enjoy are not generally the result of improvements in medical treatment but of reduced rates of infection owing to changes in nutrition, incomes, education, public utilities and personal hygiene (McKeown, 1976). Another example where such a reappraisal has taken place is in the changing views of killer diseases such as cancer and heart disease. Once seen exclusively as biological aberrations within the victims that could only be tackled with medically oriented treatments such as drugs, surgery or radiation treatment, it is now recognised that there are large behavioural and social components to both conditions and that a broader perspective is required to stem their rising incidence in Western countries.

Economic imperatives within the health systems of developed countries and an increasing recognition of the cost inefficiencies of the 'treatment driven' medical model have also prompted the search for an alternative approach. The ballooning costs of surgical and pharmaceutical treatments, together with the increasing extent to which large sections of the population are resorting to these medical technologies and drugs while continuing self-destructive lifestyles, are seen as non-sustainable, even in Western industrialised economies.

Many of these considerations have become prominent in the philosophies and assumptions of the movement promoting what has become known as 'the new public health' (Baum, 1998; Tulchin & Varavikova, 2000). The new public health represents a

> philosophy which endeavours to broaden the older understanding of public health so that, for example, it includes the health of the individual in addition to the health of populations . . . It is concerned with finding a blueprint to address many of the burning issues of our time, but also with identifying implementable strategies in the endeavour to solve these problems. (Ncayiyana et al., 1995)

Public health opposition to the dominance of the medical model in the case of psychiatric disturbance has a much longer history than that mounted in response to the medicalisation of physical illness. It grew partly out of the wider anti-establishment feelings of the 1960s and 1970s in North America and partly out of the European tradition surrounding the philosophical and political analysis of labelling by writers such as Foucault (1965). As well as emphasising the long recognised potential of diagnostic labels to enforce social norms and to create unfortunate self-fulfilling prophecies, these critics of the medical model have expressed reservations about the tendency of this approach to convert 'problems in living' into medical syndromes (Szaz, 1991). Other arguments arising out of this philosophical tradition to be presented in relation to ADHD are that the medical model encourages mental health practitioners to hunt for biological pathology at the expense of social considerations; to make arbitrary, inconsistent and often unwarranted distinctions between 'normal' and 'pathological' behaviour; to rely on diagnostic labels that are unrealistically assumed to exist as unidimensional categories; and to emphasise biomedical approaches to treatment, even in situations where psychosocial interventions may be more appropriate.

The dominance of the medical perspective on ADHD can be seen in the various diagnostic labels that have been attached to the syndrome since its first description by Still at the beginning of the twentieth century. In the 1920s it was known as 'post-encephalitic behaviour disorder' because overactivity and impulse control problems were noticed in children who survived the great encephalitis epidemics of the period. In the 1950s the growth in knowledge of the subtle effects of head injury led to the adoption of the term 'minimal brain damage' to describe its supposed aetiology. With the recognition in the early 1960s that the disruptive behaviours characteristic of the disorder were most often *not* associated with any insult to the brain, the less aetiologically derived label of 'minimal brain dysfunction' received increasing prominence. The strong behavioural emphasis in this period soon began to be reflected in a later preference for the descriptive term 'hyperkinetic child syndrome', although the beginning of the so-called 'cognitive revolution' in psychology in the 1970s produced a growing belief that the deficits experienced by these children mainly related to the difficulties they experienced in appropriately attending to and processing information (Douglas, 1972; Douglas & Peters, 1979). This led to the increasing use of the diagnostic label *Attention Deficit Disorder*, later revised to *Attention Deficit Hyperactivity Disorder* in recognition of the primacy of the disruptive behavioural symptoms, which had initiated earlier interest in the syndrome.

The various treatments that have been offered for the condition also reflect the influence of the medical model in determining the way that ADHD is conceptualised. From the early attempts to alter the behavioural functioning of these children using dietary restrictions to the current emphasis on pharmacological treatment with stimulants, the focus has consistently returned to biological modification. As indicated earlier, the use of methylphenidate hydrochloride and dexamphetamine began in the 1930s and prescriptions for these drugs have risen dramatically in recent years, particularly in America and Australia. In Australia, for example, some states experienced a 25-fold increase between 1988 and 1993 (Valentine, Zubric & Sly, 1996) and nationally the same increase in dexamphetamine use was recorded between 1991 and 1998 (Mackey & Kopras, 2001). There has been experimentation with the use of antidepressants as potential treatments for 'hyperkinetic' children since the early 1970s (Spencer, Biederman & Wilens, 1998) and more recently there has been increasing use of antihypertensive medications such as Clonidine, Guanfacine and Beta-Adrenergic blockers (Conner, 1998). While not part of mainstream practice, both developments reflect the same medicalised view of the condition and its aetiology.

ADHD may well be the 'disease for our time' because it reflects our contradictory feelings about science and the role of scientific professionals in our lives. Our unease about the results of scientific intervention and 'unnatural' treatments has never been greater and yet we increasingly opt for instant technological or medical solutions to problems as wide-ranging as infertility, obesity, erectile dysfunction and heart disease. Popular media frequently advertise these services alongside sensationalist stories denouncing the rising recreational use of heroin or amphetamine-based 'social drugs'.

The paradox is also epitomised by the growing incapacity of the public health system to cope with the ballooning costs of conventional medical procedures and pharmacological treatments, concurrent with the rapid expansion of alternative and 'complementary' approaches within the health economy. It seems as if we embrace the advances and improved treatments that science and the medical model have offered for so long, while hankering for the non-medical approaches that seem to promise something that a deficit-based approach can't deliver.

Why is the medical model an inappropriate framework for considering ADHD?

Many of the reasons for the inappropriateness of the medical model in relation to ADHD were introduced in the previous chapter and at the beginning of this one. These points will be expanded here in order to systematically examine in more detail the failure of ADHD to meet the criteria for inclusion in such a narrow explanatory framework.

Absence of reliable biological markers

Medical conditions are assumed to be identifiable physical entities. In Chapter 2, it was shown that the medical model's requirement for a measurable biological abnormality to be present was not applicable in the case of ADHD. Even the most sophisticated of the imaging devices currently available has not been demonstrated to be diagnostically reliable and there is no existing blood test or physiological parameter that clearly defines the condition or its chemical treatment.

Ambiguity among the symptoms and difficulties in making normal/abnormal distinctions

The assumption, implicit in the medical model, that clear distinctions are able to be made between the 'pathological' behaviours associated with ADHD and the 'normal' behaviours of unafflicted children was also shown to be unfounded by our current measurement practices. Even trained and experienced observers appear to be inconsistent in identifying the 'aberrant' behaviour of children with the condition and the wide variability in rates of diagnosis reflect this inconsistency.

The child's cultural milieus and other situational factors in the immediate environment appear to be as important as any intrinsic pathology in determining diagnosis. The behaviours that are supposed to mark the condition do not represent unique and unusual examples of pathology but merely responses that are within the repertoire of all children, but that are either presented in inappropriate situations or for unusual lengths of time in those who are diagnosed.

Multidimensionality of the disorder

The medical model also requires the existence of discrete diagnostic 'categories' with clear treatment implications attached. However, it is clear from the research that ADHD does not meet this basic assumption. Evidence was presented in the previous chapter of the confounding of the condition with other common paediatric problems and of the blurred divisions between ADHD, conduct disorder, learning disability and even anxiety conditions.

Importance of psychosocial variables in predicting outcome

Much of the concern with the application of the medical model to ADHD relates to the narrowed treatment options offered by this approach. It is a well established finding that stimulant therapy appears to have very little impact on actual school achievement (Weiss & Hechtman, 1993) and that significantly better long-term outcome is achieved when pharmacological treatments are combined with psychosocial interventions that simultaneously operate at the individual, family and school level. The effect of combining treatment approaches does not appear to be merely additive. Individual components act to maximise the action of the others to produce sustainable change, even though each approach on its own might have been demonstrated to be relatively ineffectual in the long term. It is significant that the relative potency of this combination of medical and psychosocial interventions increases in proportion to the severity of the presenting ADHD symptoms. (Cunningham, 1999).

Other problems with the medicalisation of ADHD

The rush to a medical diagnosis may also compromise the capacity for positive change using psychosocial interventions. As Szaz (1961) originally noted, a medical label implies that, because the person is suffering from a sickness or disease, they are no longer responsible for their behaviour. In the language of medical sociology, once access to the 'sick role' is granted, the 'patient' is considered the unfortunate victim of his or her condition. While older children and adults diagnosed with ADHD derive some comfort from being absolved from unjustified blame, it might well be that any significant improvement requires the child to assume greater personal responsibility for their behaviour as they grow older. The passivity engendered by a medical label might be counterproductive for the resumption of appropriate levels of self-management in the individual and any improvements are assumed to result from the 'treatment' that is offered rather than from individual effort.

It is interesting to note that the traditional arguments against the 'labelling' of behavioural disorders have tended to focus on the use of medically imposed diagnoses as a form of social control. Some writers continue to talk about the 'myth' of ADHD and the invention of the label and its stigma 'to help preserve social order' (Armstrong, 1995 p. 26). In many cases, however, it is actually the child's parents who request the diagnosis. The stigma of ADHD as a psychiatric diagnosis has become less aversive, in relative terms, than the stigma of perceived parenting, educational or personal failure. Such a situation has also occurred in the case of adults with mental disorders where there is evidence that increasing numbers are 'choosing' the diagnosis of ADHD in preference to other psychiatric labels because it is considered less stigmatising (Shaffer, 1994). This phenomenon obviously makes accurate diagnosis of the 'real' underlying condition more difficult and distorts the whole therapeutic process. The same distorting effect occurs with children where clinicians sometimes have to battle to accurately diagnose less 'appealing' conditions such as autism when parents express a strong preference for the more 'normal-sounding' ADHD label (Barkley, 1998a).

Many parents do not realise that the ADHD label might be stigmatising and harmful over the long term in ways that are hardly appreciated today. As Breggin (1994) has noted, the diagnosis of brain malfunction, while seeming so common, useful and consoling today, might at a later time come back to haunt the recipient of the label. As yet there has been insufficient time to observe the full effect of an ADHD diagnosis on children's future educational and employment opportunities; however, there is every possibility that security clearances, life insurance policies and licences to operate machinery, motor vehicles and aircraft might be affected. We have known for many years that psychiatric labels suggesting neurological disability tend to be surprisingly resilient—even in the face of an apparent complete 'recovery' (Rosenhan, 1973).

Unfortunately the short-term dividends of the psychiatric label continue to hold sway for many parents and the disease mentality is beginning to impact on many of the traditional social and organisational arrangements we make for the assessment and evaluation of adolescents. It is becoming relatively common for senior students sitting external examinations to apply for special consideration on the basis of an ADHD diagnosis and many education authorities are experiencing difficulties in adjudicating these requests. Boards of education across the Western world have set up working parties to develop policy in this area and there are already many cases in which applications for special consideration on the basis of an ADHD diagnosis have been rejected by education authorities and then subsequently challenged in the courts by the student (Prosser, 1999).

Increasing numbers of young people who have been caught up in the criminal justice system are also relying on a diagnosis of ADHD as a primary mitigating factor in their defence. While ADHD has long been recognised by researchers as a risk factor for traffic infringements and car accidents (Weiss & Hechtman, 1993), as well as for prison incarceration (Eyestone & Howell, 1994; Forehand et al., 1991), it is only recently that the diagnosis has become recognised in the legal community. As awareness of the characteristic behavioural patterns that describe this condition grows among the professionals interacting with these children, an ever-expanding pool of potential 'cases' is likely to come into consideration for assessment and treatment.

In epidemiological terms the current situation may be likened to the explosion in the incidence of repetitive strain injury (RSI) in the 1970s and 1980s. While current knowledge now recognises RSI as primarily a stress-related condition, the first response of the professionals involved in treating the 'disorder' was to focus on a purely physiological cause. A diverse group of medically oriented practitioners became experts in the disease and 'treatments' ranged from wrist splints to surgical procedures and chemical medication. The eventual acceptance of the finding that a complex mix of social, psychological and biological risk factors interacts to produce the disabling symptoms has resulted in the virtual elimination of this condition from the workforce.

A similar and perhaps more relevant example is provided by the history of 'dyslexia' as a diagnostic category in paediatric practice. Physicians first tackled the problem of early and unexpected reading failure in the early 1900s and the diagnosis began appearing in a number of case reports in medical journals. The label was soon generalised from a small group of highly unusual cases to cover all children who were delayed in learning to read. As a prescient indicator of things to come in the ADHD literature, it was proposed in the 1920s that children with the condition were delayed in developing the brain asymmetry characteristic of adults. This lack of asymmetry was supposed to result in 'strephosymbolia', a term used to describe the tendency toward making letter and word reversals when reading. A whole industry in eye testing and visual–perceptual training grew up around this unsubstantiated speculation and lasted until the 1970s. Needless to say it has since been found that reversals in children who experience reading difficulty are no more common than other reading errors in this group and that these children do not appear to present with unusual hemispheric symmetry. The lesson we can take from this early example is that long and unnecessary delays in offering real help with a problem can result when medicine 'discovers' a condition first.

In the case of learning disability, most of the progress in treating the condition has resulted from being more specific in the decision making during assessment. Similar specificity seems warranted in the case of ADHD. The previously discussed lack of homogeneity within the diagnostic category of ADHD has to some extent been recognised with the division of the condition into subtypes, each possibly reflecting a distinct aetiology. It can be seen in Appendix 1 that DSM-IV, as the most recent description of ADHD offered by the APA, distinguishes between children who:

1   are predominantly inattentive
2   are predominantly hyperactive–impulsive
3   exhibit a combination of behaviours from the general categories of disturbed functioning described above.

It is increasingly being suggested that the presenting characteristics of children within each of these subtypes vary significantly. Children with attention deficits without hyperactivity tend to be more anxious and shy, more prone to academic difficulties and more likely to exhibit slow and variable processing speeds. Those who exhibit hyperactivity are more likely to have concurrent conduct disorder, to be distractible and to lack many social skills. A greater proportion of boys also tend to fall within this category. A recent community survey in Australia reported that, of the 11.2 per cent of children between four and seventeen years old who were found to have ADHD, 5.8 per cent were primarily inattentive, 2 per cent were hyperactive–impulsive and 3.8 per cent met the criteria for the combined type (Sawyer, 2000).

Such differentiation of the condition into subtypes is likely to be a continuing trend and currently under consideration are subtypes that identify children who have attention deficit with learning disability, attention deficit with conduct disorder and attention deficit with learning disability and conduct disorder.

This fragmentation of ADHD into subtypes might lead to a greater understanding of the interactions that take place among the be-haviours that comprise the syndrome, and ultimately to the identification of a subgroup of children for whom a specific biological aetiology is justified. The continuation of a broad-brush medical approach to a condition with fuzzy diagnostic boundaries and an apparently heterogeneous aetiology cannot be clinically justified.

ADHD in the USA

According to the British Psychological Society report on ADHD (1996), the proportion of children meeting the DSM criteria in the USA and Canada has ranged from slightly over 2 per cent to almost 10 per cent of the population. However, as the report states, one cannot justify placing a child's behaviour within the category of a mental disorder simply because it may deviate from the norm. The report goes on to comment on the likelihood that the introduction of the less inclusive and more stringent criteria for the DSM–IV might have an impact on decreasing diagnostic rates.

With regard to the role of stimulant medication, the BPS review points out that since the 1970s there has been extensive research reporting on the effects of stimulant medication (Hinshaw, 1994; Swanson et al., 1993). It is significant that most of these studies are concerned with short-term results and not with long-term consequences. The short-term results are generally viewed as beneficial by parents, teachers and others involved with the child since the medication is seen as temporarily calming the child down. In some cases medication enables the child to be more open to help and improves their social and educational adjustment. However, a substantial subgroup appear not to benefit and a minority show adverse responses (Rapport et al., 1994). The documented side effects (Breggin, 1999; Klein & Bessler, 1992) should not be underestimated. These include sleep disturbance, reduced appetite, cardiovascular changes, stomach-aches and headaches, irritability, tics and other nervous mannerisms, unhappiness and withdrawal. Another documented long-term side effect of stimulant medication is the suppression of height and weight gain.

While most researchers and practitioners agree that medication must be combined with other forms of intervention to promote positive individual and social interaction and academic achievement, the reality is often starkly different. As Taylor and Hemsley (1995) point out, in the USA drugs have in some cases become the only therapeutic resource. Inappropriate doses and poor long-term monitoring expose children to potentially dangerous situations under the guise of 'treatment'.

In a culture that is concerned about drug abuse but is also dependent on drug-focused solutions it might not be surprising that the link between the individual and society has come full circle. Thus there is increasing concern about the fact that a large proportion of children and adolescents in the United States have turned their prescription drugs into a commodity for sale on the street (United States Drug Enforcement Administration, 1995).

The psychiatrist Peter Breggin (1994, 1999) has been a long-standing critic of the biomedical psychiatric view of children's problems, particularly the overdiagnosing and medicalising of ADHD, which he views as driven by the joint commercial interests of government-organised psychiatry and the pharmaceutical industry. He is equally scathing of some of the claims made by the research on genetics and the human genome project in which millions of dollars is spent by federal agencies, private foundations and industry to locate genes that apparently predispose people to everything from poverty and unemployment to alcoholism and crime. Breggin believes that this 'new' research lets in the 'old' discredited thinking of eugenics, which suggests that genetic inheritance and race account for particular behaviours. As Breggin states, one of the core reasons for overdiagnosing ADHD is that it appears to offer an individual solution couched in the language of 'disease and healing' for what are in reality complex social problems.

Furman (1996), a child psychiatrist, warns of 'the American epidemic called ADHD' and refers to a conservative estimate of two million children in the US who receive medication for the condition. He is critical of the DSM-IV classification for the diagnosis of ADHD, which he regards as totally subjective since, as he says, each of the eighteen symptoms listed could be said to indicate other psychiatric conditions as well as the characteristics of normal child behaviour. Furman compares the ADHD classification with the 'situational hyperkinetic syndrome', which he states Rutter (1982) found to be of no diagnostic relevance.

Furman cites the need to control health care costs as the main driving force behind the ubiquity of the ADHD diagnosis. Both Furman and Breggin express concern at the extent to which the National Institute of Mental Health in the United States directs extensive funding towards research in biological child psychiatry, the findings of which might be used to give respectability to the medical suppression of difficult behaviours.

The huge financial gain for the drug companies is a factor not to be overlooked. Furman notes that the ADHD parent support group in the United States (known as CHADD—Children and Adults with ADD) has received significant financial and other payments in kind from drug manufacturers. Furman also points out that the journals of the American Psychiatric Association (including the DSM publications) are extensively supported by advertising from the pharmaceutical industry.

Widener (1998) has pointed out that by the late 1990s, the number of children prescribed psychostimulants in the United States had increased to approximately 5 million. She too expresses concern about the dearth of studies on the adverse effects of the long-term use of these drugs and recommends the need for greater public awareness and vigilance. Widener draws attention to the need to consider the ethical, moral and social questions in the light of such excessive diagnostic zeal on the part of medical practitioners.

Diller (1990), a paediatrician, reflects on some of the broader socioeconomic and cultural changes in the United States, which he sees as potential triggers for the rising diagnostic rates of ADHD. He cites the changing nature of the family, an underresourced educational system, the problems of managed care (private health insurance) and what he calls 'the culture of disability' as some of these triggers. As he puts it, a prescriptive approach to diagnosis and treatment serves to alleviate parents' guilt. This is a sentiment echoed by Furman, who sees the epidemic of ADHD diagnoses as an abnegation of responsibility on the part of parents and the wider community.

Diller refers to the difficulties associated with managed care that defines behaviour within a rigid system of classification in order to receive medical funding. Thus behaviour with a complex aetiology is forced into the mould of being 'targeted, billed and cost controlled'. Diller argues that the justification for this approach is the belief that a pharmacological solution will be more cost effective than therapy or other treatments.

Diller is also critical of the so-called pragmatic approach of his medical colleagues to prescribing psychostimulants, which is to say, 'it works'. Diller makes the point that while psychostimulant drugs may appear to alter behaviour in the short term, their long-term effect is poor in creating any lasting change (Rie et al., 1976). As Furman (1996) puts it, psychostimulants will have an effect on almost anyone because they suppress motor activity. Ultimately

Diller confirms the view of ADHD as 'an illness for our time'. He cites the analogy of the canary in the coalmine when he states that 'the surge in ADHD diagnoses and Ritalin treatment is a warning to society that we are not meeting the needs of our children and that adults are struggling as well' (Diller, 1990, p. 9).

The high rates of ADHD diagnosis in the United States may reflect a lack of consistency in the diagnosis, treatment and follow up of the problem. A panel convened by the National Institute of Health in 1998 to develop a 'consensus statement' on the diagnosis and treatment of ADHD found many inconsistencies (*Young Minds*, 1999a). The panel found that general medical and family practitioners make the most frequent diagnoses and prescribe medication more often than either psychiatrists or paediatricians. The panel concluded that an accurate diagnosis of ADHD remains 'elusive and controversial' and that there is no evidence that medication improves either academic performance or long-term outcomes. Instead they emphasise the need for a broader social and educational perspective to assist children with behavioural problems, and improved communication between medical practitioners and educators.

ADHD in the United Kingdom

A recent analysis (*Young Minds*, 1999) showed that National Health prescriptions for psychostimulants in the UK had increased substantially to 158 000 in 1999, a 25 per cent increase over the numbers dispensed in 1998. A total of 92 000 prescriptions were dispensed in 1997, compared with 47 000 in 1996. In 1995, fewer than 15 000 prescriptions were dispensed.

Despite this increase in prescriptions the numbers of children diagnosed with ADHD are lower than in the United States owing to the use of an alternative classification system to the American Diagnostic and Statistical Manual. Britain and Europe have used the diagnostic systems of the International Classification of Diseases published by the World Health Organization (see Appendix 2), which takes a more exclusive rather than inclusive view of the criteria for diagnosis. For example, behaviours that manifest predominantly in only one situation do not constitute grounds for a diagnosis.

In the view of the British Psychological Society report (1996), medication must facilitate long-term intervention of other modes of help, rather than playing a primary role. The report emphasises the need to address both the 'within child and within context' factors, which expand our understanding of ADHD. In this regard, the BPS report makes the important point that the behaviour inventories that are often used as part of these classifications provide 'normative and comparative data for large numbers of subjects'; however, they are less effective as accurate descriptions of the behaviour of different subgroups of the population (Reid, 1995). This point comes to the fore particularly in the consideration of the multicultural factors described below.

According to the BPS report, an increasing number of black children are being excluded from schools in the UK and the number appears to be out of proportion with the number of children on the roll (Sivanandan, 1994). The report refers to two small-scale studies of hyperactivity (Sonuga-Barke, Minocha, Taylor & Sandberg, 1993) that provide evidence that the subjective judgements of those rating the children may have an effect on the outcome. The researchers compared teachers' ratings of Asian and English children with regard to hyperactivity with more objective measures of activity and inattention in groups.

In both studies, the teachers' ratings of the Asian children's hyperactivity exceeded more objective measures of their behaviours. The Asian children who were rated as equally hyperactive as their English classmates were in fact observed in the classroom to be less hyperactive. As the BPS report states, these studies raise critical questions about the use of behavioural rating scales in a multicultural setting.

As has been mentioned earlier, there has been a shift over the past ten years from a concern with aetiology towards making the behavioural expression the defining feature of ADHD. The danger of defining children's behavioural problems in this way is that such descriptions become bound by a fragmented and symptom-laden language that does not take into account individual differences and the understanding of behaviour within the context of family and social systems. Once the context for behaviour is eliminated, it becomes easier to refer to 'populations' of children and adolescents who can all be described via a common standardised *global symptom,* that is, 'they are all ADHD'.

A sobering example of this development in the UK was the decision by the current Labour government to commission the National Institute for Clinical Excellence to explore the possibility of

prescribing trial prescriptions of psychostimulants to large populations of children diagnosed with the 'combined type' ADHD,
inattention, hyperactivity and impulsiveness. It appears that the
assessment of the cost of this mass prescription at approximately 44
million pounds constituted the main deterrent to the government to
proceed with the project (*Young Minds*, Nov/Dec 2000).

The rationale for such an enquiry resonates with the view of
British psychologist Billington (1996) who identifies what he calls 'the
shift in the twentieth century from physical hygiene to the complexities of mental hygiene' (Billington, p. 40). Thus the thinking behind
the UK government initiative described above suggests a conviction
that we can 'inoculate' large populations of children and adolescents
against the expression of particular behaviours in the same way that
we can inoculate them against rubella or whooping cough.

Hill (1996), while advocating a selective use of psychostimulants
in certain cases, cautions nevertheless that such treatment should
always take into account the developmental needs of the child. He
says 'there is a risk that if Attention Deficit Disorder and Hyperactivity is understood simply as a brain disorder, other factors such
as the child's insecurities or parent's lack of support may not be
addressed'.

Child psychiatrist Davies (1996) cautions against viewing ADHD
as a single disorder. She states that its varied presentation reflects a
range of different causes. Davies echoes the American concern about
the role of government in supporting pharmacological solutions for
complex behavioural problems because parental counselling and
psychotherapy are seen as more labour and cost intensive.

Finally, McFadyen (1997) makes the point that the concept of
ADHD does not in itself suggest either aetiology or treatment. Many
of the children who come to be diagnosed with ADHD have
different personal and behavioural journeys towards this eventual
diagnosis. By medicalising the problem, it is removed from its
developmental and social context. This in turn influences the way in
which professional support and help is organised. Once the problem
is located in the child, the field of intervention narrows, since the
aim is to dispose of the problem rather than to understand it.

McFadyen states that the evidence suggests that ADHD is in fact
not just one disorder but what she calls 'the final common path' for
a wide range of behavioural difficulties that have their origins in a
multitude of factors. These may be genetic predisposition or peri-
natal factors (close to the time of birth) such as infant prematurity,

poor quality of early attachments and major stressors in the environment. If this view is correct, then it follows that an exclusively medical focus is too limiting and that professionals need to provide multidisciplinary services that reflect the complex nature of the problem.

ADHD in Australia

The first national survey of ADHD in Australia was reported in the National Health and Medical Research Council report (1997). The report provided guidelines for the diagnosis of ADHD, which included recommendations for a multi-modal approach to treatment. The report also noted some of the longer term implications from the point of view of long-term health, education, welfare and justice issues. The report's specific emphasis on greater coordination between agencies and disciplines has been most difficult to implement and little in this area appears to have been achieved. This might be due at least in part to the tendency among practitioners to give primacy to an individually based biologically driven model. As Prosser (1999) states, this trend leads to a position 'which blames individuals and their families, leaving environmental, economic, social and political influences unexplored' (p. 4). Prosser is also critical of the growing pressure in Australia to categorise ADHD as a disorder or disability, labels which he argues are inherently 'simultaneously biological and social'. The identification of ADHD as a category of disability or disorder could further reinforce a solely biological and medical response.

Since the late 1990s when the National Health and Medical Research Council report was published, there has been increasing disquiet about the high numbers of very young children, under five years of age, who are prescribed psychostimulants. An article in the *Sunday Age* (Shine, 2001) describes a survey conducted by the Murdoch Children's Research Centre in Melbourne that confirmed anecdotal evidence that more psychotropic medications were being prescribed for very young children. This despite the fact that there is no clear evidence that these drugs are at all effective for young children. A particularly disconcerting finding of the survey was that many psychiatrists and paediatricians felt under enormous pressure from parents to prescribe behaviour altering drugs. In some cases drugs were prescribed for young children that were entirely contraindicated for their particular problem.

In response to these concerns, Hazell (2000), writing for the Australian Early Intervention Network for Mental Health in Young People (AusEinet), discusses appropriate guidelines for professionals who are concerned with ADHD in pre-school children. The report concurs with the views expressed by the National Health and Medical Research Council of Australia (1997) and the Australian Psychological Society (Garton et al., 1997) that the child's behaviour must be understood within an age-appropriate and developmental context and that close cooperation with parents is an essential part of the assessment process.

Broadening the assessment process

One of the particular concerns about a purely medical approach to children with attentional problems centres on the limitations of the medical assessment process itself that in the main utilises a one-dimensional model related to identifying 'illness'. Such a model, by its very nature, ignores the complexity of interpersonal and family relationships, and also the need to understand the developmental status of the child.

The British Psychological Society report emphasises the need to obtain as comprehensive a picture as possible of the child across different contexts. These contexts include the neuro-biological as well as environmental factors such as life events, parental care, school experience, cultural background and individual psychological differences. As Whalen and Henker (1996) state, ADHD can be viewed as both a heterogeneous and a pervasive category. This means that each child has a constellation of problems that is unique to themselves and thus 'multiple domains' of functioning come to be affected and must be taken into account.

The BPS report further emphasises that what matters is the quality of information obtained in order to plan intervention. This concurs with Barkley's view (1987) that behavioural ratings, despite their apparent objectivity, are 'simply quantifications of adult opinion'. For the purposes of educational or clinical practice, they can only provide a starting point for more thorough assessments. Meaningful assessments must reflect the complexity of multiple causations of behaviour and how these interact with factors in the environment. Significantly, the BPS report concludes that assessment and planning is most successful when it involves the children themselves as active participants in the process. We take this issue of the need for children's involvement further in our later chapter on recommendations.

The need to acknowledge a multiplicity of factors as part of the assessment process is acknowledged by Hazell (AusEinet 2000), who refers to the generic guidelines put forward by the American Academy of Child and Adolescent Psychiatry for the assessment of ADHD in pre-school children. We believe that these guidelines should be part of good practice for the assessment of all children who may be considered to have this disorder. The guidelines recommend that multiple sources of information be used and that both parents be actively engaged in a partnership with the assessment team, even in circumstances where parents are divorced or separated. The assessment process should also throw light on the quality of interaction between the child and other family members through the process of observation. Useful data might also be obtained by observing the child's behaviour and interactions in the home or school environment. Hazell places particular emphasis on the need to maintain a developmental perspective in assessing the child. This includes taking a thorough developmental history with details of the child's physical, cognitive, social and emotional development. The family's social environment, family, medical and psychiatric history should also be taken into account.

This is an approach supported by Jureidini, head of the Department of Psychological Medicine at the Women's and Children's Hospital in Adelaide (2001), who points out that when children express difficult behaviour this often communicates that all is not well in the child's life. He is concerned that a rapid rush to an ADHD diagnosis because of parental pressure, limited mental health and welfare resources and lack of time can result in many deeper problems being overlooked.

One clear theme that emerges from all the discussion about the need for assessments of higher quality and depth is that all professionals involved with children, adolescents and their families, including general medical practitioners and paediatricians, require more intensive and systematic training in, and understanding of, child development.

The need for a wide range of professionals to work collaboratively, both in the assessment phase and in preparing a treatment plan for the child and the family, represents the cornerstone of a multidisciplinary approach. However, the success of such multidisciplinary work depends on an acknowledgement of child development as the centrepiece of this collaborative approach. How we can understand the nature of developmental challenges for children is the subject of the subsequent chapters.

4

Risk factors for the developing child: A psychodynamic approach

Earlier we stated that a major dilemma for clinicians and others working in the field of ADHD is the fact that individuals who receive the same diagnosis do not appear to represent a homogeneous group. However, this does not detract from the reality of everyday observations of children in schools and in early learning facilities, an increasing number of whom appear to have difficulties in concentrating, settling and following instruction. These concerns are echoed by parents within the home environment, who are disturbed by their children's antisocial behaviour, disruptiveness and, at times, escalating aggression.

The underlying premise of this chapter is that for the vast majority of children the cluster of symptoms generally associated with an ADHD presentation represents a breakdown in a complex chain of events and experiences that operate on a number of different levels. These are:

- intra-psychic—the inner world of the child, including the child's fantasy;
- interpersonal—the relationship between the child and his or her parents and family;
- psychosomatic—the link between the child's biological constitution and vulnerability to outside stress;
- social—the child's capacity to develop relationships and a life outside the family;
- educational—the child's potential for and curiosity about learning;

- environmental—the capacity of the family and the community to meet these needs.

As McFadyen (1997) has stated, the diagnosis of ADHD for many children represents a generic arrival point or final common pathway that belies the complexity and eventfulness of their journey. As described above, this journey is by its very nature a developmental one and it makes demands on the child, the family and the community. This chapter will outline how disruptions to these various developmental processes, as well as to the links that need to be made between these different levels of experience, can lead to the constellation of symptoms that we have come to associate with an ADHD presentation.

Attention as part of relational experience

This chapter introduces a psychodynamic perspective to contribute to the understanding of ADHD as an illness for our time. The psychodynamic perspective offers a conceptual framework that positions intra-psychic development, interpersonal development and the psychosomatic experience of the child as integrated processes. The successful negotiation and integration of these processes is in turn dependent on what Winnicott (1965b) has described as 'the facilitating environment'.

We will outline what we mean by a psychodynamic approach to behaviour and go on to examine the psychosocial issues that make ADHD specifically an illness for our time. The corresponding impact of these changes on children will be described.

The account in Chapter 2 of a neuropsychological approach to ADHD has given a detailed description of attention as a product of brain function and brain structure. In presenting the psychodynamic approach, our focus shifts to understanding attention as part of a relational experience, which has its origins in the earliest infant–parent interaction. We will explore potential ruptures and deficits experienced by the infant and young child, and what impact these may have on the child's capacity to later develop and maintain attention.

All behaviour has meaning and is a communication

This is a central tenet of the psychodynamic approach. It suggests that all behaviour has a goal, and that there is no such thing as aimless or meaningless behaviour. For children this is primarily the goal of creating a relationship with their parents. Professionals working in family therapy who use a family systems approach, which suggests that changes in one member of the family can affect other family members, would suggest that all behaviour has to be seen within a context. The psychodynamic approach emphasises that behaviour always has a context, both in terms of the child's inner world fantasies, hopes and fears and their response to everyday outside pressures. For example, parents may be angry and irritated by what they perceive to be the destructive behaviour of their child—but this behaviour is nevertheless a communication. Understanding that *all behaviour has meaning* allows us to view attention in a different light, so that we see it not simply as a cognitive activity but primarily as a relational response that emerges out of the earliest attachment and bonding experiences between the child and their parents.

The events surrounding our infancy and childhood shape our future

A psychodynamic approach suggests that our earliest experiences in life affect our future development. It takes seriously the importance of our early experiences and the major impact that these have on later life. A simple example of this would be to ask oneself whether as a child one vowed never to repeat a particular word or phrase that one's parents had used. However, now as a parent we may find ourselves not only using the same word or phrase but using exactly the same intonation! It is particularly important to keep this in mind when we think about describing the child with ADHD as parents may identify similar problems in themselves as children. While there may be some organic or biological connection in these cases, we should not overlook the fact that the *patterning* of emotional and social relationships can have a profound effect. The capacity and indeed the tendency for people to repeat particular patterns of behaviour are very powerful. For example, a woman who was very concerned about her three-year-old boy's hyperactivity seemed to find it difficult to attune herself to what her little boy was trying to communicate. Interviews with the family revealed that he was a very anxious child struggling to make emotional contact with his mother. His mother in turn had had a very restricted, rigid upbringing in which expression of emotion was barred or often misinterpreted. We can suggest that she actually lacked a repertoire or any preparation to know how to receive the communications that her child was making. Her husband, in contrast, was more emotionally in tune with his son and did not agree with his wife's 'diagnosis' of their son as hyperactive. The way he put it was 'she wants you to give her the manual that will help her to work the child'.

Ultimately a psychodynamic approach allows us to explore the fact that the child is always more than the presenting syndrome and is a timely caution against the tendency to describe children through a diagnostic category. Instead it can help us to understand how problems such as ADHD might reflect a variety of complex inter-relationships within the family and in the family history.

Behaviour is dynamic and not static

Another facet of the psychodynamic approach is the emphasis on behaviour itself as dynamic and not static. In fact, behaviour is seen as changing all the time. By seeing the child as more than a syndrome we open up an opportunity for communication rather than closing it down. In this approach, *timing* can be critical. We can thus question why a child behaves in a particularly aggressive or attention-seeking or demanding way, or why his behaviour suddenly becomes overactive. This does not deny that the behaviour is genuine and can be distressing to the family and people who are trying to deal with it. However, a tendency to dispose of the behaviour or to immediately search for a strategy might paradoxically be misleading and will foreclose on our need to gather more information about the *meaning* of the behaviour for the child and *the context* within which it occurs.

The timing of the presentation of a problem can give us an important clue as to what a child may be feeling. For example, the presentation of overactive behaviour and a persistent lack of concentration might mask a more deep-seated depression or intense anxiety brought on by particular events in the life of the child or young person.

Adrian, a six-year-old boy, was referred for an assessment following concern in his primary school about his poor levels of concentration, inability to sit still and disruptive behaviour. His teacher was convinced he had ADHD and various strategies were put in place that focused entirely on managing his behaviour in the classroom. However, at the assessment it was clear that much more lay behind Adrian's behaviour since he had been brought up in difficult and at times traumatic circumstances before being fostered by his parents at the age of four. By taking a developmental history it was possible to understand the meaning of Adrian's behaviour within the context of his life experience. This indicated that his intensive activity was a way of covering up his high level of anxiety about separation and loss and about being abandoned.

The overt and the covert in behaviour

The psychodynamic approach recognises that unconscious processes have a role to play in how we both construct and sustain attention. This extends the field of enquiry beyond the immediate behaviour or symptom that is presented. We are able to consider that the child's inner fantasies, their dreams, their capacity for play and the content of the play are all data that can throw light on the child's behaviour and place it within a context that is unique to their emotional environment.

For example, a child may be very disruptive in the classroom, have a poor attention span and be unable to complete a task. Our contact with the family may reveal that there has been some serious disruption in the family such as an acrimonious separation or a problem of a more chronic nature. In situations such as this, the child literally might not be 'free to use their own mind' on school-related activities, because their main preoccupation is with the family problem, which they are unable to solve. Broadening the field to include unconscious processes also enables us to recognise that in some cases the symptoms of ADHD actually have a specific defensive function. For example, continual overactivity might serve as a protection for the child against the terror of being overwhelmed by feelings of panic, fear and depression. A constant state of activity and disruption can be useful if it prevents one from having to be alone with disturbing thoughts. This was clear in the case of Adrian, who had lived with a psychiatrically ill and alcoholic mother before being moved to multiple foster parents before the age of four.

When Adrian commenced therapy he was almost entirely verbally silent, but engaged very actively and imaginatively with all the toys in the room, which represented a different dimension of communication. Adrian in fact went to 'the heart of the matter' in his play with the doll's house. Here he would repeatedly seek out the mother doll and push her head viciously down the toilet bowl. On some occasions she would be stuffed into a cupboard. From time to time cars and trucks would find their way into the doll's house, riding over the occupants and smashing all the furniture. Through his play we could begin to understand his rage and confusion about the mother who had mistreated him and then dropped him as well as his fear that he could lose the safety of his current home at any time.

We can thus see that what might be described as disruptive or difficult behaviour might actually have a protective function for the child and be used to enable them to process overwhelming events in their lives.

Is ADHD an illness of our time? Risk factors for the developing child

The following account of some risk factors for the developing child and adolescent attempts to provide a social context for an understanding of the emergence of the behaviours that have come to be associated with ADHD. These risk factors are primarily associated with the increasing numbers of children who are 'diagnosed' with ADHD for whom this presentation might be indicative of a variety of other problems and causations. We do not include in this group those children who present with 'pure' ADHD, for whom 'brain insult' or dysfunction clearly leads to recognised attentional deficits. Our primary concern is with the uncritical expansion of this diagnostic category to describe children whose problems need to be understood as part of a complex and interactive experience.

In presenting the risk factors below we attempt to expand on what has been described as 'the social landscape of childhood' (Polakow, 1992). This inevitably includes the daily lived experience of children, for example in the institutions of childcare, school and in their experiences with their parents.

We are not suggesting that there is a direct causality between any one of these factors and ADHD. Rather, we hope to change the emphasis of much of the current thinking about ADHD, which searches—mistakenly in our opinion—for a direct cause and effect.

As Jureidini (2001) puts it, the problem with the search for an apparently and deceptively simple solution is that it is usually wrong. We hope to show how the child's behaviour emerges instead out of a complex chain of interrelationships that provides the biopsychosocial context of development.

Speed of change and the difficulty with managing time

It has become a platitude to state that the only thing that can be guaranteed is change itself. As individuals we experience change at an unprecedented level in all aspects of our family, social and economic life. Nevertheless there is a tendency, for the sake of maintaining a sense of security, to behave as though everything is still the same. Obvious changes that have been wrought in family life in the past 40 years include the changing role of women and mothers, the high divorce rate and the very fact that families can take so many different forms. However, for families struggling with the day-to-day realities of caring for children, there is little support to help them to accommodate these changes. For example, the lack of connection between work and family life leads in many cases to stop-gap arrangements being made for children, which compromises attention *for* the child.

The uncertainty about the availability and duration of work itself and the all-pervasive anxiety about workplace changes inevitably have an effect on the way in which family life itself is constructed. The most significant change is in the lack of time itself. Those who have employment are often working significantly longer hours, with weekend and evening trading blurring the distinction between work time and recreation or family time. Many women and mothers discover that a greater personal liberation has not led to a greater sharing of the responsibilities for the day-to-day care of children. In many cases they are burdened with having to juggle two jobs, one at home and one in the workplace. The coining of the term 'time poor' gives us some indication of the profundity of this change. Domestic help, home management and even the everyday care of young children become areas of activity that require to be 'outsourced'.

Growing up in a 'multimedia' environment

The bombardment of information through the multimedia makes it extremely difficult to learn how to discriminate between what is useful and important and what is not. Children find it extremely difficult to know not just *how* to, but also *where* to allocate attention. The area of electronic information is one in which parents find it hard to set the rules since often their children's knowledge and skills in this area have already overtaken their own. The image of the 'sound bite' promoted by television also suggests that attention is a fleeting process that must be capitalised on before the viewer becomes bored and switches elsewhere.

Social disadvantage

Deficits of attention within the community exist where many long-term unemployed families and some single-parent families experience a lack of choice and opportunity. This keeps them in the grip of poverty and, over time, alienates them from a sense of investment in society (Pugh & De'Ath, 1984). In Britain the term 'socially excluded' is used to describe these families. For these most vulnerable families and children the environment does not provide a facilitating experience. Instead of receiving greater attention to meet their needs, they have in fact borne the brunt of cuts in health and welfare services and the depletion of educational resources. For these families, their social exclusion becomes a chronic state of mind that leads to the cycle of deprivation on all the intersecting levels described at the beginning of this chapter: the intra-psychic, interpersonal, psychosomatic, social and educational.

Lack of 'attentive presence'

The deficits of attention described above and the changes to the very nature of time management that have been brought about in the broader community through socioeconomic and technological change do not sit well with the specific time frame that parents require in order to assist the child to develop appropriate attention. This is a time frame in which the pace should be set by the child. It is a time frame that is essentially linked to the parent's *attentive presence* and availability to develop a *partnership* with the child that is based on the understanding that parents cannot be made at birth but *become parents over time through trial and error.*

The parenting task is one that must involve fathers as well as mothers. In fact, underestimating the role of men and fathers might be particularly significant in the aetiology of ADHD. Are we, for example, to assume that it is purely coincidental that the number of boys who are referred for ADHD exceeds that of girls? We know from our clinical practice and from life experience that the mental health of children is as dependent on fathering as it is on mothering and on the use of good authority.

Decline of the extended family and the sense of community

The fragmentation in many cases of the extended family and the lack of a sense of personal community and continuity also have a major impact on the fabric of family life and the development of appropriate attention. The concept of an emotional ecology springs to mind, which suggests that children thrive in environments that acknowledge the interdependence between different aspects of experience such as home and school, family life and work, rather than environments in which these experiences are split off from each other. The process whereby this takes place is one of *containment*, where the containment provided to parents through extended family, friends and community enables them in turn to provide containment for their children.

Countries such as Australia, the United States and the United Kingdom have a history of migration and the experience of migration inevitably involves a reassessment of the ideas, values and traditions that have been handed down from previous generations. Parents might be separated physically from their countries of origin as well as from the values and traditions that provide them with containment. In some cases they might feel that these values and traditions are no longer applicable, in a changing world, to the rearing of their children.

These many changes leave us in a state of transition. We cannot parent as our parents did but we have not yet arrived at a new place so we are somewhere in between and floundering. The anxiety generated by such uncertainty can lead to a demand for increasingly mechanistic and oversimplified solutions for extremely complex problems. The identification of ADHD as an umbrella diagnosis for a wide range of behaviours might be a prime example of this dilemma.

The erosion of childhood

It is becoming increasingly difficult in a consumer-oriented technological society to acknowledge the real dependence of children and the fact that children have infantile needs and require a time frame of development that takes cognisance of this developmental fact.

The sense of urgency of rushing through childhood might reflect the needs of some parents for their children to be independent and self-sufficient as soon as possible. This might lead the child to develop a compliant but false independence that belies the brittle and vulnerable person beneath.

As has been mentioned earlier, contemporary parents often have very high expectations of their children, which does not leave much room for trial and error, or the inevitable failures that are also an important part of the learning process. The concrete thinking involved in the current pragmatism that all problems must have a solution or strategy also prevents children and young people from *learning from their own experience.* If we take this attitude to its logical conclusion it leads us to a position in which children's behaviour requires to be *managed* rather than *understood.*

Long-stay childcare

We acknowledge that the provision of good childcare is an essential part of the support that needs to be made available to parents in bringing up their children. The accessibility of good quality child-care is a great boon to parents and many childcare environments offer interesting, stimulating experiences for children. However, we need to be mindful as well of the long-term effects of long-stay childcare on children, particularly at the critical stages of their development from infancy through early childhood, when the capacity for attention requires an optimum environment for its development. Findings from a number of studies (McGurk et al., 1993; Ochiltree & Edgar, 1995) suggest that the *quality* of childcare is the critical factor in ensuring a positive outcome for children. Vandell and Corasaniti (1990), in their longitudinal study, found that at eight years of age children who had been exposed to poor-quality day care as infants were rated by teachers and parents as having poorer peer relationships, emotional health and school work habits and as being more difficult to discipline than children who had been reared in part-time childcare or exclusively at home.

The question of what constitutes quality care is one that clearly needs to be addressed. In the interests of children and their mental health, it is also one that needs to be viewed outside of political, financial or other vested interests. One way of beginning to do this

67

is to consider what the experience of childcare might really be like for the child.

Traditionally, childcare research does not concern itself with the specific observation of children and with analysing their experience since 'outcome' is based on the views and responses of those people who are outside of the child, namely the child's parents, carers and teachers. Including an understanding of the child's lived experience introduces scope for a more three-dimensional enquiry into the impact of childcare. This could also prove to be a rewarding area of multidisciplinary collaboration.

Observing the child's lived experience

The detailed observation of infants and young children as a field of study has developed within a number of different settings. First, it has been used in the clinical setting as a preparation for therapeutic training (Miller, Rustin, & Shuttleworth, 1989). Second, it has been a catalyst for change, as in the ground-breaking films made by the Robertsons (1989) on the observation of the impact of separation and loss on young children. Finally, observation has come into its own in field research within the social sciences. Polakow (1992) provides a compelling observational account of what she describes as 'a modern institutional childhood' through a two-year study of five childcare centres in the American Midwest.

Polakow's observations of the social and interpersonal context of the childcare institutions makes disturbing reading. The inclusion of a number of privately run centres in the sample gives us a taste of things to come in Australia, where deregulation has been more recent. Polakow's main thesis is based on the assertion of the educationalist Donald Vandenber that the ultimate aim of childhood as a life phase is 'a becoming at home in the world' (Vandenberg, 1971, cited in Polakow, 1992). Play is the main mode through which this realisation takes place. The child 'restructures, invents, makes history and transforms reality'. However, in Polakow's analysis of the child's experience within the different childcare centres, she found little understanding of this process. Instead she found that staff, although well intentioned, appeared uneasy with free play and sought instead to make the children's stay as 'productive' as possible, by imposing a series of activities that had 'adult-centric agendas'. Her account throughout is of the standardisation of children's experience, particularly through what she describes as the 'socialisation of institutionalised time'.

With regard to the children's behaviour, she found confusion in staffing attitudes towards aggression. This would lead some to be 'laissez faire', while others took an overly rigid stance. This in turn led to an increase in aggressive behaviour among the children. In the worst of the private centres, large numbers of children were cramped into limited space. The high turnover of poorly paid and poorly trained staff led to a fragmentation of the interpersonal relationships surrounding the child, which should have constituted the cornerstone of the child's experience.

As Polakow points out, the task for the child to 'become at home in the world' is a formidable one. For a modern child in the West it is particularly complicated. This is due in part to an overanalysis of the child's experience by competing social scientists, all vying for 'theoretical ascendancy and prescriptive power over a generation of parents and teachers who have surrendered their powers of "knowing" and "seeing" to the professionals . . .' (Polakow, 1992, p. 22). We return to the ways in which these powers of 'knowing' and 'seeing' can be reinstated for parents and professionals in Chapter 8, where we explore new paradigms for helping children, parents and families.

The physical setting: life in an open-plan world

At many childcare centres children live for long hours in what is an open-plan world. It is not unusual for some children to be placed in childcare at seven in the morning and collected at six or six-thirty in the evening. In fact, there are now opportunities for parents to place their children in childcare centres over the weekend. The difficulty for children in maintaining themselves within the open-plan space is that there is no wall or separate room and no sense of privacy, which means that no boundary can be established between themselves and others.

Here, the structural and social setting literally fails to help the child to develop sufficient attention in order to begin to differentiate between themselves and other people. In other words, to know where their body boundaries end and others begin.

In the United States, Lally (1995), director of the Center for Child and Family Studies at the Far West Laboratory in California, has emphasised the need for policy-makers to understand how the day-to-day childcare environment influences the infant and young child's capacity to establish what he calls 'identity formation'. He states that, 'never in history have so many young children spent so much time in the presence of non family members'. He is critical of what he calls the childcare *industry*, which can become little more than a *minding environment* for children, where both the status of the task of caring for children and its remuneration is severely under-valued. Lally refers to the 'explosion' in the numbers of children in childcare in the United States, which means that infants as young as five or six weeks of age can be found in infant care and that these arrangements are commonplace for six-month-olds. Lally makes the point that these infants and young children are at a critical stage of their development, since they are in the process of developing 'a working sense of self'. The caregiver's responsiveness and capacity to understand this process is essential.

Where caregivers are insufficiently trained and have to care for large numbers of children, it is inevitable that they might fall back on ways of protecting themselves from emotional pain and a fear of becoming too close to the child by 'not becoming too attached'. However, it is of course precisely this attachment that the child requires in order to grow and flourish, since the caregiver is, in Mahler's (1985) words 'the outer half of the child's self'.

Lally, in line with Polakow, is critical of the training that many childcare staff receive, with its focus on the establishment of routines, rather than on the development of relationships. He refers to the work of Mosier and Rogoff (1994) who have shown how infants learn about their potency or its absence through the success or failure of their relationships with their caregivers, and their use of their caregivers as instruments to achieve their goals. Thus the day-to-day, minute-by-minute interrelationship between child and caregiver is, in Lally's view, not simply a cognitive event but forms the building blocks for the child's development of a core sense of self.

Lally draws attention to the increasing concern in the United States about the 'quiet crisis of infant neglect', which has led the Carnegie Corporation to launch a major national initiative to assess the impact of the scarcity of high-quality care.

Childcare as an 'industry'

Deregulation has led to an increase in private childcare facilities, which means that the care of young children becomes increasingly dominated by the profit motive. The long-term implications of turning the care of young children into a business initiative might yet need to be assessed. McGurk (1997), in his analysis of the use of the term 'childcare industry', questions whether this change is purely linguistic or whether it reflects the power of language to shape the way in which social issues are construed. As he puts it, to speak of childcare as an activity gives primacy to the needs of the client group, whereas to talk of it as an industry shifts the focus towards the economic aims of those activities. McGurk questions whether the best interests of children can be served by an industrial or commercial orientation to the provision of childcare.

The lack of a quiet environment

One of the problems of an open-plan environment where there is little attention to the personal space and individual needs of children is that the noise level is often very high. This factor in itself can preclude the possibility of the child developing attention skills. The pioneering work of psychologists Vygotsky (1962) and Luria (1961), which explored the process by which attention develops in children, is particularly relevant in this regard. They identified subvocal or *inner speech* as the precursor for the development of self-regulation in children. In order for this process to take place, it follows that the child must find himself in an environment in which he can literally 'think his own thoughts'.

The question of how children develop attention and language skills is presented in some interesting research by Ward (1995, 2000), a speech pathologist specialising in attention and language development in Manchester. She found that an unusually large number of children were referred at an early age for language delay and language difficulties and wondered how this had come about. In an analysis of 1000 children, she found that one in five had listening or attention problems that delayed their language development. As a speech pathologist, Ward believed that language is a key factor in the development of attention because language provides the child with the mastery of being able to make sense of the world, and of being able to both gain and give attention.

In her analysis of the children in the study, she found that they did not suffer from developmental delay. Rather, the problem lay with the high level of noise in many of the households in which they lived and the lack of attention they received from their parents. In many of the households the television set was left on all day as a background noise and as a result the children were often unable to discriminate between significant communications. Ward also noted that the parents in this group appeared to have very little actual verbal contact with their children apart from the brief times related to getting them up in the morning and putting them to bed at night. In response to this problem, Ward put in place a language program whereby the parents were actively encouraged to talk with their children. This involved them having to sit down in a face-to-face interaction with the child for specific periods in the day. Ward found that these simple language exchanges had positive results within a short space of time.

In addition, Ward found that many of the mothers in this sample were nervous about using baby talk or 'motherese' because they believed it would encourage dependency in the child. Of course, Ward and other researchers in the area of infant mental health have pointed out that exactly the opposite is the case; that baby talk or motherese is not only the baby's way of getting attention but forms the most fundamental foundation for the development of language. Murray and Trevarthen's (1986) study of the role of the infant in mother–infant communication found that the mother's baby talk was an adaptive response to the communication elicited by the infant. Their findings confirm the reciprocal nature of these communications and the importance of the infant as an active initiator.

Murray and Trevarthen go further in stating that their findings suggest that these infant capacities elicit in the mother a complementary 'human environment', with the mother augmenting and elaborating the child's limited capacities for self-regulation, feeding back affectively toned responses that the child 'assimilates'. They propose that the infant's satisfactory development requires this complementarity.

Attention and discontinuity of experience

Two other researchers, Bain and Barnett (1980), point to the difficulties that might emerge for children in long-stay childcare where the staff might not have sufficient training and understanding of the nature of child development and the way in which children learn to develop attention. They were involved in an Action Research Project in a family day care centre in Britain. In the course of their study they observed that the staff placed considerable focus on routines, which appeared to take precedence over the needs of the children and over the relationships that they had with the children. They observed that when the children were occupied with a particular game or activity they would be interrupted in an arbitrary way and moved on to another activity. Bain and Barnett described this interruption from the point of view of the child as a *discontinuity*, where an experience is suddenly cut off and not followed up at a later stage. Bain and Barnett found that where there was a series of such discontinuities in the course of a day, the children in the group who had a tendency towards aggression became more aggressive and difficult to handle, while the children in the group who might have had a tendency to be rather timid became more withdrawn. Thus the discontinuities of experience in themselves appeared to damage the children's capacity to develop appropriate attention.

While most researchers would agree that quality of care is a major factor, there tends to be less agreement about what actually constitutes quality care and how best this can be achieved. Longitudinal research on child care, such as that carried out by The Early Childhood Research Network (2000, 2001), may throw light on these complex issues by identifying the relationship between child care and variables such as a child's cognitive development and capacity for emotional relationships.

The emotional landscape of childhood: The loss of play and its implications

The concept of discontinuities of experience throws light on the importance of play for the young child and its role in developing the capacity for attention. In an ever more competitive environment, the anxiety of parents for their children to succeed has led to the establishment of early learning centres that suggest a more formal environment in which play has either been superseded or has become very task oriented. Parents on kindergarten management committees increasingly demand what they refer to as 'product' from the children and their carers in the form of artwork or other visible signs that the child is 'learning something'. Parents recommend in some cases that children spend less time on individual activities and be rotated through a variety of activities throughout the day, so that they can produce more at the end, in what appears to be a factory assembly line approach to play.

Despite the fact that these recommendations are well intentioned, they are based on two fundamentally incorrect assumptions about the meaning of children's behaviour. The first is the assumption that the activity *in itself* has a meaning for the young child. In fact, the child only begins to engage in an activity if it is appropriately mediated by a caring and supportive adult. In other words, the child learns to engage with activities and becomes curious about them *through a relationship.* The second is the assumption that unstructured play that the child initiates themselves has no meaning and therefore no intrinsic value. However, it is through apparently unstructured play that children actually successfully learn.

The reason for this is that play for the young child represents an experience that can be simultaneously serious as well as fun. It is also real work, since play enables children to negotiate the boundary between their inner fantasies and fears and the realities of the outside world. Play also offers unique opportunities for problem solving and for the development of social relationships.

The capacity for play that involves the use of fantasy thus provides a foundation for cognitive development and for the child to begin to engage in higher levels of reasoning and abstraction. The capacity to play also offers protection for mental health, since it enables the child to play out 'the worst scenario' in a way that can make it seem less threatening and more manageable.

Clinical experience suggests that children who present with severe attentional difficulties often find it hard to engage in imaginative play. Their play instead tends to have a limited and repetitive quality. They find it hard to be selective when offered the opportunity to play with a range of toys and quickly become overwhelmed, choosing to mix and mess up the toys or declare their boredom after trying something once. This behaviour suggests that these children have not been able to develop the capacity for play as a process that can help them to take a step away from themselves and assist them to make sense of painful and difficult events. Instead, their inability to play and tendency towards mess and destructiveness suggests a state of inner persecutory anxiety.

The need for early childhood workers to develop a greater understanding of the importance of play for children and of how to link this with a 'play based curriculum' is emphasised by Walker (1999). She carried out a study of early childhood programs selected randomly from a cross-section of centre-based care and sessional kindergartens in metropolitan Melbourne. Staff completed a questionnaire about their current practices regarding opportunities for the children in their care to play indoors and outdoors, the way in which transitions and routines were handled and whether structured or unstructured artwork was promoted.

The responses indicated that the vast majority of children in the sample were engaged in a predominance of large-group rather than small-group activities. There were many and lengthy 'mat times' for the children when they were expected to sit still and listen to a story or join in a song. Art activities focused in many cases on following ready-made designs and the opportunities for free and informal play were limited primarily to indoor activities.

Growing up in a female world: Denial of differences between boys and girls

It is generally acknowledged that boys from infancy through at least to adolescence are primarily looked after by women. We do not stop to think of what impact this might have on the need for boys to be able to identify with a male role model. It is not uncommon for many boys at an early stage of their development in childcare centres, in kindergartens or in the early levels of schooling to be identified as having deficits of attention or for teaching staff to 'request' a diagnosis for ADHD. Often these boys will be described as misbehaving, aggressive or unable to settle to a particular task.

However, in making this kind of snap diagnosis it is important for us to consider that we might be misinterpreting the behaviour of boys who might well be struggling to find ways of communicating with their parents, teachers and caregivers. What is often described as attention seeking might in fact be an attempt to seek closeness and intimacy. However, the way boys might choose to go about trying to make this contact is very different from the way girls might go about it. Boys use their bodies differently in a more vigorous interaction with the outside world. This is not necessarily an act of aggression but may become so when it is not understood within its context and responded to appropriately.

Sinason (1992), a child psychotherapist who has worked extensively with children and adolescents with mental disabilities, makes the comment that the use of the term 'attention seeking' is one of the greatest abuses we can visit upon children, first because it dismisses their behaviour as meaningless and second because children are justified in seeking attention as an essential requirement for their emotional survival and the development of a sense of self.

A more appropriate and less reactive response to the behavioural problems presented by boys in early childhood centres and later in the educational system would be to act preventively. This would involve the provision of appropriate male role models for young and adolescent boys. It is a sad reflection on our time that fewer men are prepared to enter teaching as a career, particularly at primary school level, because of the threat of litigation concerning physical contact and child abuse (Caroline Jones, *The Age*, 1999). Paradoxically, it is an *increased* presence of good supportive male role models working in partnership with women in early childhood settings and in the schools that would make children less vulnerable to abuse.

The impact of separation and divorce on the developing child

It is another well known fact that the divorce rate in the Western world has been on the increase for years. In the United States, which is said to have the highest divorce rate, 40 out of 100 first marriages end in divorce compared with 16 out of 100 in 1960. The divorce rate for second marriages is about 10 per cent higher than for first marriages (Karr-Morse & Wiley, 1997). This sheer weight of numbers and our tendency to view divorce as the norm might lead us to view its effects on the family as a 'lifestyle' change rather than as one that will have major implications for the child's future development.

When parents themselves are struggling with the aftermath of ending a marriage or partnership there is a tendency to overlook the difficulties that children might be experiencing, which might lead to a pretence that nothing very important is happening. This façade of matter-of-factness, which is defensively assumed by many children and their parents, has the potential to break down at a later stage with damaging consequences. The recognition and validation of the child's experience and the containment of the child's pain are vital elements in helping both the child and the parents *to process* the experience.

> Two parents requested advice late on a Friday afternoon about how to tell their young children that the father was leaving the home the following morning. He pointed out that he had *already* placed his suitcases in the hall. In these circumstances one could only inform the parents that they would be confirming what the children already knew.

The idea that 'children don't know what is going on' is one of the most prevalent in child-rearing. It leads to justifications about keeping children uninformed and unaware, which in turn promotes high levels of anxiety in children. These states of anxiety might quite understandably lead to lack of concentration and disruptive behaviour in children.

In research carried out in the UK by Cockett and Tripp (1994), direct interviews with the children themselves elicited some striking findings. For example, only a small minority of children—one in sixteen—stated that they had been prepared by their parents or informed by them of the impending divorce and separation. Mothers in these circumstances claimed that their children were 'too young to understand' and only informed the child of the separation after their partner had left the family home.

The children whose families had been what the authors described as 're-ordered' through separation or divorce were more likely than children from intact families to have encountered health problems, especially psychosomatic disorders, to have needed extra help at school, to have suffered lower self-esteem and to have experienced friendship difficulties.

The outcomes were generally worse for children who experienced three or more different family structures than for those living for the first time with a lone parent or in a stepfamily. These children were more likely to describe themselves as 'often unhappy or miserable'.

Fewer than half the children in re-ordered families had regular contact with the non-resident parent, usually their father. Half of the children did not know where the non-resident parent was living.

Children who had experienced a series of family disruptions were not only less likely to have contact with the non-resident parent but also received less support from extended family networks.

The absence of fathers and fathering

The findings of the above study on the impact of separation and divorce are particularly significant in that they identify the problem of the absent father. This might be useful to enable us to create a working hypothesis about the consequences of family disruption for the psychological development of the boy. While the next chapter goes into this aspect in more detail, we might here consider some of the broader psychosocial consequences. As has been mentioned previously, we need to understand why a substantially larger number of boys are referred for ADD and ADHD diagnoses. While not wishing to suggest a direct correlation between divorce and ADHD, we nevertheless need to consider the struggle for the developing boy in the absence of a supportive male role model or presence.

The relationship of children to parents of the same sex and different sex form the emotional building blocks of life. These relationships ebb and flow and go through many changes, not least of all because the child requires different types of support and identification from each parent at different times. As we have stated previously, development is dynamic, not static; it changes all the time. Thus, for example, a boy's perception of his father and his need for his father's presence at the age of five are different from what they would be at thirteen. For boys whose fathers have no contact with the family, this poses a painful problem.

We must, however, be mindful of the fact that the absent father might also exist within the family in which there is no separation or divorce. In these families all of the emotional life is centred on the mother while the father absents himself emotionally or physically through demanding hours of work.

In the United States, Blankenhorn (1995) describes the social consequences of an increasingly fatherless society as declining child wellbeing. He states that our society is 'unable to sustain or even find reason to believe in, fatherhood as a distinctive domain of male activity'. Blankenhorn believes that the role of fatherhood has been radically diminished by men's loss of a specific role and loss of authority within wider society.

By contrast Blankenhorn believes that fatherhood is in fact society's most important role for men. Fatherhood, he says, 'more than any other male activity helps men to become good men; more likely to obey the law, to be good citizens and to think about the needs of others . . . Fatherhood bends maleness—in particular male aggression toward prosocial purposes' (p. 25).

Blankenhorn's view of the importance of the role of the father is echoed by Widener (1998). She observes that in clinical work with so-called ADD/ADHD children, there is often a continuing problem of an absent father. She refers to Breggin's comment (1994; 1997) that the condition could be renamed DADD (Dad's Attention Deficit Disorder), because in many cases the father's absence is the underlying cause of the child's acting-out behaviour. Breggin states that a caring and loving relationship with their father is an effective curative factor for many children with behavioural problems.

Widener quotes Strean (1997) who comments on the dynamics underlying the absence of the father in child-rearing. Strean identifies several clinical characteristics of how the father has been experienced by adult patients in later life. These are

> a tremendous emotional hunger for the father experienced as being absent during childhood. Many men and women feel anxious and fearful to depend on, or be intimate with a man. Many men have an emotional inhibition due to the expectation of being emotionless which has been taught from infancy onward. Because of this emotional inhibition many fathers are passive and withdrawn except when showing anger. (p. 276)

This last factor becomes particularly relevant when we consider the place of both parents in setting appropriate boundaries and limits for the child.

The loss of good authority—the importance of setting boundaries and limits

One of the major issues of our time is the confusion between being authoritarian and using authority. As parents, professionals and educators we wish to move away from a Victorian mode of bringing up children in which they were seen but not heard and often tend to the other extreme of an inability to use authority appropriately, and becoming laissez faire. At the core of this anxiety lies a fear of being negatively construed; parents fear the hatred of their children and teachers fear the negative feelings of their pupils or indeed of parents. However, a psychodynamic approach takes the view that setting limits and having appropriate boundaries is an essential part of containment and demonstrates to the child our care and concern. Thus, paying attention is intrinsically linked to giving attention and receiving attention, which in turn can only emerge out of appropriate and containing structures where good limits are set and boundaries acknowledged via an *enabling authority*. These structures ideally need to emerge out of more creative partnerships between the family, the school and the surrounding environment. This allows children to know where they stand and thereby have the freedom to grow and thrive.

For example, in the case of Adrian it was important to engage in a collaboration that extended beyond Adrian and his parents to include the school. It was fortunate that Adrian's teacher was prepared to attend some joint meetings where we could discuss Adrian's behaviour in the classroom. For example, Adrian's hypervigilance about changes to his environment was evident when he became particularly unsettled when computers were installed in the classroom. Understanding the meaning of Adrian's behaviour enabled the teacher to move beyond a list of disciplinary actions to more realistic and flexible limit setting. This proved to be extremely helpful for Adrian, who felt contained and understood by his teacher. It also set him on the path to demonstrating his considerable academic skills. Most significantly, the joint endeavour enabled the teacher to recognise that he too was being heard and supported, which made him less anxious about Adrian and therefore enhanced his own capacity to act effectively.

The use of good authority thus sets the scene for the important developmental task of *containing anxiety*, a task that runs like a leitmotif through all of the developmental stages and is an essential prerequisite for the development of attention.

In conclusion, an understanding of children's problems within a family and social context moves away from a position that identifies the problem as existing solely within the child. Moreover, an acknowledgement of the wide range of external risk factors for children further justifies a multidisciplinary approach to children's behavioural problems and in particular to ADHD. In the next chapter we take further the developmental process for the child in relation to their parents and show how this goes hand in hand with the capacity for attention.

5

The capacity for attention and the developmental process

In this chapter we develop the view that attentional problems have their origin in infancy and early childhood. Our focus is therefore on this crucial period of development.

Developing attention in the infant

The capacity to develop attention has its roots in the earliest infant–parent relationship. The famous paediatrician and child and adult analyst, D. W. Winnicott (1965b), made the point that 'there is no such thing as a baby'. By this he meant that the infant and the personality of the baby develop within a context. Thus the infant's development takes place within the framework of social embeddedness. It exists within a relationship with the mother, father, family and significant others. This kind of social and emotional embeddedness suggests that the beginning of life, that is to say relational emotional life, actually takes place before the baby is even born. The baby is 'held in mind' by both parents for nine months, through their ideas, thoughts, fantasies and worries about him or her. The term that Winnicott has used for this process is *maternal reverie*. This emotional preparation for the infant represents a particularly important kind of attention, since it has both a biological and an emotional function, for mothers as well as fathers. The capacity for reverie might be interrupted by depression in one or both parents, anxiety arising out of financial difficulties, poor marital relationships and a variety of other factors.

Winnicott (1965b) also states that 'the baby looks at the mother and sees himself'. Infants make up a picture of themselves and how they appear by scrutinising their mother's face and expressions and responding either to the joy and delight in them or to her depressed or inverted gaze, her anger or her inability to understand what effects these produce physically or emotionally. Researchers in the infant mental health field refer to the baby's capacity to hold a gaze as a useful way of initiating the process of attention. Even at this very early stage of infant development we can identify babies who are not able to sustain attention since they have not reached the first stage of being able to hold a gaze. This problem is striking, for example, in observing babies who suffer from a failure to thrive, which suggests that the fundamental holding relationship between infant and mother has not yet taken place.

The reciprocal and hopefully rewarding interaction between infant, mother and father is viewed by a variety of clinicians and researchers in the field as a fundamental precursor for the development of attention. Sameroff and Emde (1989) describe how 'attention emerges out of relatedness and the infant and young child's relationship with significant care givers'. Stern states that 'the infant comes into the world bringing formidable capacities to establish human relatedness. Immediately he is a partner in shaping his first and foremost relationships.' He goes on to say: 'The infant's first exposure to the human world consists simply of whatever his mother actually does with her face or with her body or hands. The ongoing flow of her acts provides for the infant his emerging experience' (Stern, 1977, p. 33 and p. 9).

The emphasis on a dynamic partnership between the infant and their parents is particularly crucial and is referred to by Trevarthen (1979) as 'the proto conversation'. This emphasis on partnership is further amplified by Klein (1967) who asserts that our language for describing the foundation for attachment and bonding needs to move away from an emphasis on the *ego* and the individual self to what he calls *'we go'*, which connotes a more vigorous partnership between the baby and their caregivers.

Bowlby and attachment theory

John Bowlby (1973a, b & c) is best known for introducing a new perspective to thinking about the nature of the relationship between mother and child through the comparison of human young with that of other animal species. This research led him to conclude that attachment is as necessary for emotional survival and mental health as food and shelter is for physical survival. Bowlby saw attachment as deriving not so much from the feeding relationship itself but from physical closeness that allows intimacy between the mother and the baby to develop. He identified five innately-based patterns of response between a mother and baby. These instinctive patterns are intimately linked to the giving and receiving of attention. The baby initiates contact with the mother by sucking, clinging, crying, following and smiling. These serve the function of linking the child and the mother and of obtaining her care and protection in return. Such early attachment relationships serve to construct a 'psychological map of the world' for the developing child. This internal representation consists of objective (cognitive) as well as emotional (affective) knowledge of the world. Sameroff and Emde (1989) refer to this process as laying the foundations for 'the centrality of affect and shared meaning' between the child and the caregiver.

Operationalising a model of attachment—the strange situation test

Bowlby's original ideas on attachment, separation and loss have led to research carried out in Britain and the United States on how infants and their mothers and fathers actually cope with everyday separation and loss. Ainsworth et al. (1978) have operationalised these ideas through the development of the Strange Situation Test. In order to ensure object constancy, the test is carried out with babies between the ages of twelve and eighteen months. In the test, the baby and mother are observed together to establish their normal patterns of interaction. The mother is then asked to leave the room and the baby spends a short period of time with the observer. When the mother returns to the room the quality and type of interaction between mother and baby is observed. A number of different categories of attachment are described that most clearly fit the quality of the infant and parent interaction upon reunion.

Ainsworth and her colleagues carried out research across different cultures, and came to identify three main categories of attachment:

- secure attachment
- anxious–resistant attachment
- anxious–avoidant attachment.

Secure attachment is characterised by the infant who can respond positively to their mother's comfort on reunion. The anxious-resistant baby might allow the mother to comfort them only intermittently while the anxious-avoidant baby might actually withdraw from the mother and seek to comfort themselves.

As attachment research has developed into its 'second generation', a fourth category of attachment has been identified by Main et al. (1985), which is known as the 'disorganised category'. This category is most typified by infants who have experienced serious abuse and neglect. Ainsworth's research suggests that these early patterns of attachment provide diagnostic indicators for subsequent adjustment to parent–child interaction. The research has implications for understanding the earliest diagnostic signs of the beginnings of attention problems. We can thus see that the mother who cannot attend to her baby sufficiently to contain their anxiety already begins to set up a pattern of response in the child where they believe that their needs might be met only intermittently.

ADHD as a problem of containment

The child's experience of attachment and the parent's availability to bond with the child can also be expressed through the dynamic concept of *containment*. This is a concept originally developed by the British psychoanalyst Wilfrid Bion (1964). Bion described the early infant–parent relationship as personified by the process of 'the container and the contained'. Here the parents are the containers and the baby requires to be contained. This process of containment enables the parents to transform the negative or anxious communication of the child so that it becomes reintegrated in the child as a tolerable experience. Where the parental caregiver is not able to provide this containment the child is left with undigested anger, despair or feelings of persecution that cannot be transformed into more tolerable states of mind.

Essential to the process of containment is *the capacity of the parents to tolerate anxiety and uncertainty,* that is at times not knowing what is happening to the baby. This is particularly important since it enables parents to take the time to observe their baby directly, and to be cued by the baby rather than rush into solutions that might not be appropriate. The concept of containment and the capacity to tolerate anxiety is intrinsic to the paradigm of emotional ecology referred to in Chapter 4. The reason for this is that the work of containment cannot take place within a vacuum: the mother needs to be contained by her partner, the parenting couple needs to be contained by family and friends, and the community as a whole needs to value the task of parenting.

This concept of the container and the contained is particularly useful in attempting to understand the presentation of ADHD, since the typical characteristics of inability to settle to a task, flitting from one activity to another and distractibility indicate behaviour that is quite uncontained. We might hypothesise that the child is literally not able to be alone with their own thoughts because they are too anxiety-provoking and that the containing processes and inter-actions in their life in the form of parental support might either never have taken place or might have broken down.

The development of the capacity to be alone as a precursor to the development of attention

For the child, the capacity to be alone is an essential prerequisite for learning and cognitive activity, of which reading is the most obvious example. While we might assume that this ability comes naturally, it is in fact dependent on finely tuned interactive processes that take place at a very early stage in the child's emotional development.

> Adrian, who we discussed in the previous chapter, had great difficulty developing a capacity to be alone. We have referred previously to his hyper-vigilance. This was something he employed in the home even in the presence of his devoted foster mother. She was not allowed to close doors and had to let him know in advance when she was going to hang out the washing, which meant that she would be outside. When Adrian played in the front garden on his own or with friends, he could not bear to have the front door closed.

Winnicott's earliest writings (1965) foreshadow the problem of ADHD when he describes one of the tasks of the young child, particularly as they begin their experience of learning and settling at school. This is the task he calls *the capacity to be alone*. This is a signif-icant milestone in the development of attention. In order to learn to read, and to be able to take in information, the child has to be able fundamentally to be alone with their own thoughts. Winnicott describes the capacity to be alone as originating in the experience of the young child who *is able to be alone in the presence of another*, for example, the child's mother. Winnicott states that the child needs to be able to play, to dream, to be near their mother or in a place or situation that represents her care without constant reference to her or without the need for constant interaction. The child needs in a sense to be able to 'forget' their mother for a short period while they become engrossed in activity. Earlier on, we referred to the difficulty some children have in concentrating on schoolwork because they cannot forget the tensions at home, and they remain deeply preoccupied with unresolved problems from their core relationships.

In conclusion, from the perspective of early infant development, the ability to develop attention is part of a complex learning process that is dependent on the effective and mutually rewarding relationships between the infant and their caregivers.

Developmental biology and current infant research

American clinicians and researchers Sameroff and Emde (1989), as we have indicated earlier, perceive the infant–caregiver relationship to be of supreme importance in providing what they call 'the centrality of affect'. That is to say that the child's emotional state and awareness emerge out of this central relationship, which is the cornerstone of all developmental and cognitive experience. Sameroff and Emde make the point that the repetition of experience—that is, its continuity—has more impact than a single experience. This is borne out by clinical experience of seeing families whose problems are often repeated across the generations. Unless these families receive support and understanding, problems will be repeated in the next generation.

Sameroff and Emde also emphasise that far from being the blank slate waiting for something to happen, the infant is already biologically primed for interaction. This idea of the baby as an active partner in interaction with their caregivers is very important for the way in which we view ADHD. We tend to talk about it as though it exists solely in the child and has little relationship or meaning within the context of the child's relationship with their parents or significant members of the family.

Emde (1987) describes the five basic inborn motivational principles in the infant–caregiver relationship. These are:

- activity: the baby's developmental agenda
- self-regulation: the baby's capacity to manage emotional hazards and environmental perturbations
- social fittedness: the baby's capacity for behavioural synchrony and a partnership with parents
- affective monitoring: the baby's capacity to discriminate pleasurable and unpleasurable experience
- social referencing: the baby's capacity to pick up emotional/ social cues from caregivers.

In referring to a developmental agenda Emde makes the point that the baby's activity is centred on emotion and relationships. This enables the baby to make developmental gains and also has a biological function in that the interaction between the infant and their parents promotes a level of activity that increases neural firing in the central nervous system. This leads to increased connections between neurons or brain cells, so that systems of increasing complexity come into play.

The infant already has a capacity to handle emotional hazards so that development at all times is goal-oriented or task-oriented. Emde traces a parallel between the infant's capacity to manage emotional or environmental perturbations and the biological capacities of the cardio-respiratory and metabolic systems. Above all, the infant seeks out a way of fitting in; thus the infant has a biological need to make sure that their behaviour synchronises with their parents. This is carried out by both emotional and physiological means through eye contact, gaze and in turn by the parents' capacity to pick up cues from the child and intuit what they need.

Emde confirms the importance of baby talk, which has biological, neurological, social and emotional functions (Snow, 1972) and refers to the work of Papousek and Papousek (1979), which underlines Murray and Trevarthen's 1986 findings that the parent equally has a biological readiness to relate to the infant. Examples of this would be the parent's exaggerated greeting responses and imitation of the baby's facial and vocal expressions. In ideal circumstances infants and parents 'mesh their behaviours in delicately timed mutual interchanges' (Sameroff & Emde, 1989). Trevarthen uses the term 'protoconversation' to describe this fundamentally interactive relational experience between the infant and mother which becomes in effect the foundation for all subsequent social interactions.

Emde refers to social referencing as the infant's way of being in touch with their caregivers. Again we see how this is dependent on an interactive process as opposed to something that happens to the child in isolation. Thus the availability of the parents sets up a pattern of emotional signalling between parent and child that is central to the child's subsequent growth and development.

Bio-behavioural shifts and developmental transformations

Emde (Sameroff and Emde, 1989) states that development is not a linear experience but one that is subject to change and transformation. This links with the basic tenet of a psychodynamic approach that we described earlier: of behaviour as dynamic, not static; constantly changing. Emde describes bio-behavioural shifts and periods of change and transformation as operating on the level of the *psychosomatic*, the *affective* and the *cognitive*. These shifts have important implications for the emergence of a number of different developmental skills and capacities in the infant and young child. They typically take place at two to three months, six to nine months, approximately one year and at eighteen to 21 months of age. These periods of transformation also come to represent 'stage boundaries in cognitive development' (Uzgiris, 1976).

Bio-behavioural shifts also comprise critical shifts in socio-emotional and perceptual motor development. Emde states that the very wide-ranging nature of these bio-behavioural shifts or changes in the infant and young child lead to the hypothesis that they reflect significant regulatory shifts in the central nervous system.

The connections between emotions and developmental transformations

The close interaction between biological changes in the child, their social environment and their emotional state is demonstrated by Emde's observation that the child's affective changes most typically come at the end of a shift. This heralds a new level of biopsychosocial organisation for the child and sets the scene for further developmental consolidation. These emotional or affective changes in the child, such as smiling, or stranger and separation anxiety, are in turn critically dependent on the feedback the child receives from the parents and lead to their internalising the experience of change as positive or negative and to their added sense of mastery.

How can these ideas be applied to children with ADHD?

The work of Emde and others in the field of infant mental health (Fraiberg, 1980; Stern, 1985; Sameroff & Emde, 1989; Sroufe, 1989) confirms the central position of the interactive relationship between the infant and their caregivers as a core organising principle for the development of positive mental health. This interactive relationship provides the infant with what is simultaneously a process and a structure. Thus, when caregivers hold the infant in mind they create a space, which enables the infant to begin to think for themselves. We might hypothesise that the child with ADHD lacks a *core internalised* holding parent, around whom they can organise their thoughts and actions. The reasons for this are undoubtedly very complex. They might be related to constitutional factors such as the baby's vulnerability at birth or feeding and settling difficulties, which would be sufficient to interfere with the finely tuned interchanges between the infant and their parents. They might also derive from the readiness of the parents to parent, the state of mind of the mother at the birth of the child, the marital and parenting relationship and the quality of the external supports available.

Emde makes the point that the outcome for children becomes problematic when the caregiver's emotional availability is not satisfactory. He states 'the organising role of affect in its dual aspects—i.e. the simultaneous monitoring of emotional signals from oneself and from others—can lead to developmental problems'. Thus for children with ADHD symptoms there might be a confusion in the emotional signalling process whereby there is insufficient monitoring of emotional signals *from within the self* in the sense of Vygotsky's 'inner voice' and an ignoring or misinterpretation of the emotional signals received from others. At its most fundamental this represents a failure in the ability to organise or integrate emotional and cognitive experience.

The development of the 'inner voice' and the ability to monitor and interpret emotional signals, which is so dependent on the early relationship with a responsive caregiver, was a problem for Adrian. Throughout all his sessions he maintained a particular facial expression, which at first sight resembled a wide grin. However, as this appeared to be his sole facial expression, it came to take on the appearance of a permanently fixed grimace. Adrian's facial expression alone hinted at the huge strain he experienced in attempting to suppress his confused and anxious feelings about his past life and his fears of being dropped again in the future He had difficulties making and keeping friends. In the playground, he would cling to one child and hit out at others if they encroached on this friendship. This inevitably led to his becoming isolated because the children became wary of his possessiveness.

How can we identify problems in early childhood?

The conclusion that the period of infancy and early childhood is critical to development leads to questions about how to identify the particular developmental trajectories that might lead either to adaptive or maladaptive outcomes. Shaw et al. (1996) explored the risk factors in the period of infancy that lead to disruptive behaviour in early childhood, and concur with the view expressed by a number of clinicians and researchers that 'much of what we know about the predictors and correlates of early disruptive behaviour suggests that there are multiple pathways to the same destination'. They refer to previous research (Richman, Stevenson & Graham, 1982; Rutter, 1978), which indicates that families from lower socio-economic backgrounds experience more risk factors overall from a variety of sources or 'multiple domains'. They also refer to research that has shown that poor infant attachment has been significantly related to later externalising problems, particularly among groups of high-risk children (Erickson et al., 1985; Shaw & Vondra, 1995).

Their own findings confirm the critical importance of the period of infancy in that disorganised attachment status, maternal personality risk and child-rearing disagreements were found to be predictive of later disruptive behaviour problems. At a broader level they also refer to the cumulative impact of a number of stressors over time in the period of infancy and how these can determine the developmental trajectory of child behaviour.

The link between postnatal depression, anxiety and ADHD

One of the stressors consistently referred to in the literature is that of the mother's depression. Shaw et al. (1996) refer to studies that indicate a close link between the mother's depression and the child's later disruptive behaviour (Fergusson, Lynskey & Horwood, 1993).

Other studies have shown that children with disruptive behaviour problems have mothers who report more depressive symptoms (Mash & Johnstone, 1983).

In our clinical experience we find that many of the children who present with ADHD also experience considerable underlying anxiety, often to the point where they are literally tormented by fears of attackers or the wrongs that have been done to them. In these cases the heightened anxiety and activity of the child often exist in striking contrast with the depression in the mother, compounded by her sense of weakness and hopelessness. It might be suggested that the mother's depression is a direct result of the child's overactivity. However, this conclusion would limit our understanding of the problem since it would return us once again to the position of viewing ADHD as existing solely within the child and denying the interactive nature of the problem.

Research on the impact of postnatal depression on development

Murray's (1992) longitudinal research on the impact of postnatal depression on development has thrown light on the specific ways in which the infant and young child are affected by the mother's depression and how this in turn influences the child's subsequent development and capacity for learning. The research explores how different kinds of mother–infant interactions are associated with different kinds of developmental outcomes.

Murray followed up a sample of women and their babies over a period of eighteen months following the birth of the child. On the basis of a screening for depression, the women were divided into two groups—those with a previous history of depression, that is depression that preceded the pregnancy and birth, and those women who had become depressed after the birth of the baby. The infants in both groups were assessed on a number of cognitive tests as well as on the Strange Situation Test.

The results of the research are significant in pointing to the way in which specific cognitive functions were affected by the mother's depression postnatally. The research found that the children of mothers whose depression occurred with the onset of the birth, that is those women who suffered from postnatal depression, had a poorer outcome than those children whose mothers suffered from depression prior to their birth. This would suggest that the circumstances surrounding the birth and the mother's possible ambivalence about having the child were significant factors in the aetiology of the depression. In addition, the findings showed that the mother's depression resulted in a much poorer outcome for the boys in the sample and made them more vulnerable. The research findings suggest that if the mother's depression was related to marital difficulties, the negative feelings towards her partner could flow on to ambivalence towards her son.

Murray's findings concur with the research findings mentioned earlier, particularly the finding that maternal depression following the birth of a child exacerbates the effects of other variables that may already exist, such as lower social class and limited language development. This confirms, as we have mentioned before, the need to be aware of the existence of a wide range of psychosocial factors that come into play in exploring the aetiology of behavioural difficulties in the child.

Depressed mothers' speech to their infants and its relation to infant gender and cognitive development

A further aspect of Murray's research showed that the mother's depression had in some cases a quite devastating effect on the quality of communication with their infants, particularly their male infants. In particular there was an impact on language and emotional tone in these interactions. We have referred previously to the vital function of baby talk or motherese. Stern (1985) has described the critical function of the mother–baby speech pattern leading to core relatedness. Trevarthen (1979) uses the term *primary intersubjectivity*.

In her research, Murray found a tendency for depressed mothers to relate with greater hostility and criticism towards their boy children. This appeared to affect their cognitive development, since by eighteen months of age these boys performed less well than the girls on the cognitive tasks. As Murray explains, if this was combined with a less favourable environment overall, then they were even further disadvantaged.

Longer term follow up

The children in the sample were followed up five years later (1995) by Murray. In a variety of constructed play situations the five-year-olds were asked to show what happens in their families at important moments—mealtimes, bedtimes, bad and favourite times. The observations were then rated according to different dimensions such as care and control by parents, neglect, aggression, marital relationship and the child's ability to give a verbal account of the play. The children's narratives were also subjected to a linguistic analysis. The results showed that children of mothers who experienced postnatal depression were less likely to view themselves as a character taking action and initiating events, and were more disposed to using negative constructions to talk about their experiences. The impact of the mother's depression on the child remained significant even though in some cases the mother had overcome her depression. Murray further found that at five years the boys were more likely to be behaviourally disturbed, hyperactive and distractible, while the girls tended to be overly concerned with the needs of others.

Maternal depression and the ADHD child

In her research, Murray discusses what she calls the potential for greater irritability of male infants in the general population, which makes greater demands on the mother and requires a greater level of responsiveness on her part. Murray's findings point to the poor longer term outcomes for boys whose disadvantage on a number of levels might start at birth. These findings might throw some light on the disproportionate number of boys who are referred for ADHD. Murray's research does not make any mention of the fathers in the sample, and it would be interesting to know more about their involvement and its possible mitigating effects.

The finding of the lower cognitive results overall for the boys in the sample gives us an indication of the many aspects to the problem. These might range from learning difficulties through to behaviour problems and their existence affirms the importance of maintaining a strong multidisciplinary approach in our attempts to find solutions.

The development of a flexible, integrated child as opposed to an anxious, brittle personality

It is not uncommon for parents to report concern about their child's aggression or angry outbursts together with other characteristics of the child's personality that might be designated as a symptom of ADHD. Sometimes the aggression is described in terms of the child damaging things or of a lack or concern or care for other people. In presenting a psychodynamic approach to the problem we suggest that the containment and understanding of aggression in children as well as in adults is central to understanding development and also throws light on the meaning of this disconcerting or difficult behaviour.

The critical task for young children as they progress through the different states of development is to be able to negotiate intense feelings of love and intense feelings of hate, often simultaneously. These emotions are not exact opposites but rather complement each other and are a normal part of all development for children and adults. As we have mentioned earlier, our society demonstrates confusion about these experiences and tries to deal with the confusion by creating a split between loving and hating. This results in the difficulty associated, for example, with the use of *appropriate authority* in setting boundaries for children, for fear of being thought *authoritarian*. However, the task for parents is not to edit out aggression or dispose of it but rather to contain it.

In Winnicott's classic paper on the subject of hatred, he puts forward the proposition that 'a mother has to be able to tolerate hating her baby without doing anything about it'. The reasons a mother hates her baby are numerous according to Winnicott. Among them is the fact that the baby 'is ruthless, he treats her like scum, an unpaid servant, a slave'. The baby is also a threat to the mother's physical state, her private life and her own personal pre-occupation. The point that Winnicott makes in presenting these challenging ideas to parents is that we need to recognise that the mother's hatred for the baby, as well as her love for the baby, is an inextricable part of normal development. In good circumstances the mother's feelings towards her baby can be acknowledged, held and *contained safely*. This can enable the baby in turn to experience their own sense of hateful feelings towards their parents in a safe way, which acknowledges the reality of what the baby feels. Winnicott's description of the early infant–parent relationship is a vigorous one, which is the antitheses of a *sentimental environment* in which strong emotions are denied.

We need to understand that the developmental tasks of early childhood are extremely intense and take place at a rapid rate for the child. Recognition of the child's feelings and the child's real emotional experience—that is to say taking their emotional experience seriously, is integral to helping the child to negotiate the ability to deal with hating and loving feelings, which in turn helps them to begin to develop the inner resources that are so necessary to their later psychosocial development. However, for parents this cannot take place in a vacuum. In order for them to support the infant and young child, they too need to feel supported and contained. This suggests an emotional ecology in which there is a clear inter-dependence between individual development and social and environmental factors.

> Martin, a twelve-year-old boy, had been assessed as having ADHD and was prescribed psychostimulants by a paediatrician. However, the paediatrician felt that Martin and his family would benefit from therapy in view of the parents' concerns about their son's wild temper tantrums. On assessment it was clear that Martin's problems were of a very longstanding nature and perfectly illustrated McFadyen's concept of ADHD as the 'final common pathway' for a multitude of problems. An only child, Martin had difficulty differentiating himself from his parents, in the sense of knowing who was the parent and who was the child. His father was away from home for months at a time, and while he was away Martin assumed control of the house, a situation to which his mother acquiesced. Through his absence, Martin's father became a longed-for but increasingly tantalising presence. Martin's plans for what he and his father would do together on the latter's return were always dashed because of his father's lack of commitment to a fathering role. Although about to start secondary school, Martin had never succeeded in sleeping alone in his room and had slept with his parents since birth, a situation his mother had encouraged in view of her husband's long absences. It was not surprising therefore that Martin raged against his parents during the day when they so clearly failed to help him at night to overcome his infantile anxieties and terrors and develop more effective inner resources.

The rightful place of depression and anxiety in child development

Depression and anxiety equally represent important emotions and experiences that both children and parents have to negotiate as part of normal integrated development. Each contains within it components that provide a link between our inner world experience of hopes and fears and the outer world. For example, depression can be seen as an opportunity to provide a more effective mode of thinking, to integrate our experiences and literally to digest what we have learnt and heard. Anxiety too is necessary for the developing child to feel that there is sufficient challenge to prompt them to move into the next stage of their development. By this we do not mean challenging the child to do things before they are ready or creating artificial stress situations, nor are we suggesting that children should be encouraged to be depressed.

Rather an awareness and recognition of anxiety and depression as *potential growth points* helps children to develop inner resources. Here we come full circle because the management of deeper and more complex emotions also sets the scene for the child to begin to maintain appropriate attention. This leads them to begin the process of learning and relating to other people and to becoming aware of other people's needs. It is also a process that leads to the flexible, integrated child rather than the anxious, brittle personality. However, children can only develop these resources, that is the capacity to negotiate depression, anxiety and frustration without resorting to instant aggression or destructiveness, when they know that the adult world has an investment in promoting this awareness. Thus children develop these resources through relationships, whether it is with important caregivers or the people who take the place of caregivers, such as childcare staff, kindergarten teachers, sports instructors, school teachers and others.

Essential to this process is the capacity of caregivers to validate the child's experience. Emde (in Sameroff & Emde, 1989) stresses the problem for the child whose painful life experience can be what he calls 'disconfirmed' by the caregivers around him who deny the factual reality of the painful experience as well as the opportunity for the child to express their feelings about the experience. This produces what Winnicott (1965a) has called 'the false self'. In this uncertain state the child does not have permission to *attend* to their real needs and their *capacity for attention* thereby also becomes compromised.

6

The concept of self-regulation: Creating links between a neuropsychological and a psychodynamic approach

What is the common ground between the neuropsychological perspective and the psychodynamic approach to ADHD? Recent research and clinical studies suggest that the insights of neurobiology and the link with early infantile experience might provide a promising start. These findings lead us to change our focus from viewing ADHD as a distinct syndrome to viewing the condition as the symptomatic outcome of a highly complex interrelationship between the development of brain structure and the actual experience of the child.

Rima Shore (1997) suggests that we need to replace our 'old thinking' about the brain as developing in a linear mode with 'new thinking' about the brain that indicates that there is a complex interplay between genetic endowment and the experiences we have. These experiences have a significant impact on the 'architecture of the brain' that in turn affects the activity of the brain. She points out that by the time children reach the age of three, their brains are twice as active as those of adults. Most significantly, the early interactions of childhood create not only a context for development but 'directly affect the way the brain is wired'. Of particular significance is the recognition that for infants and young children there are *prime times* for acquiring different kinds of knowledge and skills.

The concept of self-regulation

Allan Schore (1994) sees *the regulation of affect* or emotional experience as a cornerstone of this connection as well as the necessary goal or outcome of the maturational process. Schore is optimistic that the 'phenomenon' of self-regulation might prove to be a point of convergence for psychology and neuroscience. Schore asserts that self-regulation is an essential organising principle of all living systems. As such, it is one of the few theoretical constructs that are utilised by all scientific disciplines. It is multi-level and multidisciplinary, and can be studied along a number of separate but interrelated dimensions from the molecular level through to the social and cultural level. The concept of self-regulation within the context of a developmental and psychodynamic approach is particularly useful because development itself for the child is characterised by a progression of stages in which there is a close interaction between the child's capacity to develop self-regulation and their capacity to engage with their environment.

Schore believes that close and positive contact with the caregiver is essential for the infant and young child to achieve regulation of affect through regulation of the developing autonomic nervous system. Here the self-organising capacity of the developing brain, that of the infant and young child, occurs in the context of a relationship with another self and another brain—namely the primary caregiver. The latter acts as an 'external psychobiological regulator of the *experience dependent* growth of the infant nervous system'. These experiences shape the maturation of those structural connections within the brain that are associated with socio-affective functioning.

Siegel (2001) points out that we must take into account the fact that the brain is 'a complex set of integrated systems that tend to function together'. This emphasis on integration is particularly relevant when we consider the impact of suboptimal relational and attachment experiences for the child. Siegel states that the orbitofrontal region of the brain, which is central to processes such as emotion regulation, empathy and what he calls 'autobiographical memory', might depend for its functioning on the quality and nature of interpersonal emotional communication during the early months and years of life. The quality of this collaborative and attuned communication between infants and young children and their parents establishes what Siegel calls patterns of interaction that provide opportunities for regulation of the child's positive and negative emotional experience. Thus an examination of 'interpersonal neurobiology' gives rise to an understanding of the way in which a sense of self is constructed.

Schore (1994) maintains that in 'misattuned' relational environments of parents and child, the high levels of negative emotional experience actually act as growth inhibitors for the developing brain. In cases of severe deprivation, brain development can be abnormal, as indicated by limited elaboration of connections within the brain (Kolb, 1995). As McFadyen (1997) points out, the most dramatic example of the capacity for self-regulation is found in premature infants. The immature nervous system of the infant is extremely sensitive to the external environment, which includes the mother's tuning in to her baby's physical and emotional state. The infant's capacity for, and quality of response to, their total physical and emotional environment will influence their ability to develop self-regulation. The capacity for self-regulation is particularly significant in modulating normal responses and in creating appropriate inhibitions.

Clinicians in the field of infant mental health now believe that the earliest infant–caregiver relationship creates feedback systems or feedback loops that are essential to the establishment of autonomy and self-regulation within the infant. Here we can see how the psychodynamic concept of an interactive emotional partnership between the infant and the caregiver has a parallel in the concept of feedback loops within the baby that correspond to feedback loops within the parent.

Brazelton and Cramer (1990) identify four key feedback systems that come into play. These are:

- synchrony
- symmetry
- contingency
- entrainment.

These feedback systems relate to Emde's identification of the specific innate responses within infants, referred to in Chapter 5, which are intended to elicit responses from within the parent. Thus, as we have stated previously, the infant is biologically primed for attachment and for initiating a specific communication and response pattern.

The four feedback systems referred to by Brazelton and Cramer take as their starting point the belief on the part of the carer that the baby's behaviour has real meaning and is a communication. This implies an essential interconnectedness at this early stage of life between the biological—the beginning of the workings of the brain, and the emotional, that is the meaning that is attributed to whatever the baby does and communicates. The key factor here is the capacity of the caregiver *to tune in with the baby.*

The feedback system of entrainment mentioned by Brazelton and Cramer is particularly relevant for our understanding of ADHD and of self-regulation. It is within this interactive exchange that the caregiver—mother, father, or both—meet their baby's initiative and interaction and extend and prolong their baby's involvement and attention. The capacity for play and flexibility is vital here, since it enables the baby to take turns at being in charge and to initiate their own interaction. This requires a degree of flexibility on the part of the parents, which in turn depends on their capacity to contain anxiety and not to intrude or too readily take over the infant's attempt at interaction. Thus, as has been stated before, *the baby in fact teaches his parents how to parent.*

Self-regulation and maternal depression

If we believe that the establishment of self-regulation in the infant is dependent on a mutually absorbing and sensitive interaction with their mother and father, then the parents' state of mind and their own capacity for attention is a critical part of this process. The depressed mother and father might not be in a position to begin this engagement with their baby. Lynne Murray's research, referred to in Chapter 5, shows us that the children of mothers who are depressed at the time of the child's birth do less well on cognitive tasks. Of particular significance is the fact that they also develop problems with sleeping and feeding and that these problems are greater for boys than for girls.

Co-regulation as a prelude to self-regulation

The capacity to establish appropriate sleeping and feeding patterns is a cornerstone of self-regulation, combining as it does biological needs within the context of the emotional and social environment. In order to achieve an appropriate state of sleeping and eating, the infant and their caretakers need to go through a process of co-regulation. The establishment of these patterns, as well as the capacity for self-restraint and self-monitoring, becomes more difficult within an inconsistent environment. Such an inconsistent environment could be characterised by the physically or mentally absent parent who *cannot hold the baby in mind*. An environment, for example, in which the infant and young child can never predict the nature of the parent's response becomes an environment in which there are diminished opportunities for emotional and social development.

The capacity to establish feeding and sleeping patterns can there-fore be said to represent important templates for development for the infant and young child that have profound implications for later behaviour. Through the feeding experience the child takes in so much more than food. Feeding depends on a mutually rewarding relationship, which already at this early stage enables the infant to construct an inner image of themselves. The capacity to establish a regular sleeping pattern makes equal demands on the infant–parent relationship, requiring as it does the ability of parents to contain their own anxiety about separation and death.

As Murray's research indicates, the co-regulatory process is critical for the infant boy, who is particularly vulnerable to incon-sistencies in the environment. The absence of a dependable co-regulatory experience with a depressed unavailable parent will therefore diminish the infant and young child's capacity to establish autonomy and self-regulation.

Self-regulation and learning problems

As we have mentioned earlier, children referred for ADHD are often found to have an overlay of learning and reading problems. Grainger (1997) describes the development of self-control as an important foundation in the capacity of the child to learn. The development of self-control and self-management are, she states, reliant on the ability of the individual to develop what is called self-guiding speech. Self-guiding or private speech has its origin in early childhood and is equivalent to 'thoughts spoken out loud' as private speech becomes internalised by the child as part of the self-regulation process.

As Grainger puts it 'the development of behavioural self-control is linked to the emergence of an internal self guiding dialogue', a concept akin to the previously described work of Vygotsky and

Luria. She goes on to say that ADHD, rather than being a pattern of failure in attentional capacity, might in fact be a lack of development of appropriate self-regulatory processes. The capacity for self-control lays the foundation for attention. The capacity to complete a task thus depends on the opportunity to have experience of *problem solving, rehearsing and expanding* the internal dialogue. This is a view that resonates with Brazelton and Cramer's four feedback systems that describe the early interaction of the infant and their parents.

The impact of trauma on self-regulation

Perry et al. (1995) in the United States describe what they call the 'neurobiology of adaptation and use-dependent development of the brain' with regard to the way in which childhood trauma is processed. Perry and his colleagues are critical of the way in which the concept of resilience is used too readily to describe children under stress. This leads to a potential denial of the fact that infants and young children are extremely 'malleable to their environment'. Perry sees the important relationship between neurodevelopment and traumatic experience in infancy and early childhood as highly significant because of what he describes as the 'plasticity of the brain'.

In infancy and early childhood the brain is at its most sensitive to all stimuli from within the body and to interaction with the outside world. As Perry states, 'experience itself is the organising framework for the infant brain at its most receptive'. Thus emotional and physical experience will actually have a structural impact on the way the brain develops. In normal brain development in the infant and young child, whatever the child experiences will trigger the development of neurons in those parts of the brain that are used to deal with that experience. Here use-dependent and sensitisation models come into play, which are also part of the normal learning process since they involve repetition.

Perry and his colleagues postulate that for the infant and young child, repeated consistent exposure to trauma, emotional deprivation and uncertainty will establish typical patterns of neural activity in those parts of the brain most associated with affect-regulation, inhibition, humour and empathy. Repetitive exposure to stress over time will elicit an *adaptive response* in the child—but one that is likely to elicit misunderstanding on the part of others and that ultimately will be unhelpful in the child's interaction with the outside world.

Perry describes significant gender differences in the way in which these responses to stress are expressed. Boys resort to a greater degree of hyperactivity and impulsivity, characteristics that may be viewed as coming under the diagnostic category of ADHD. This gives us an indication of why more boys than girls are diagnosed with this disorder. Perry states that girls have a different adaptive response to stress, one that is manifested by what he and his colleagues call 'the dissociative freeze or surrender response'. Girls internalise their problems and become depressed. This finding might also throw light on why fewer girls than boys overall are diagnosed with ADHD and indeed referred to child guidance clinics. The unhappy and depressed girl at the back of the class might never bother the teacher and might therefore paradoxically be less likely to be referred for treatment.

Perry and his colleagues' reference to 'use-dependent' and 'sensitisation models' of neural functioning in response to stress is particularly relevant when we try to understand how apparently small and meaningless events can trigger an extreme aggressive or impulsive response in a child. Perry explains this as the sensitisation of parts of the brain to stress at a vulnerable time in the child's life, which results in turn in an overresponse or an oversensitivity to apparently minimal cues. This would confirm one of the tenets of the psychodynamic approach that 'all behaviour has meaning and is a communication'. An example of this type of 'sensitivity' and the powerful impact of past traumatic experience can be seen in the following extract from the case of Adrian, whom we have discussed earlier in the book.

> Both of Adrian's parents had been alcoholics and his mother had in addition suffered from a psychiatric disorder. Adrian's foster parents knew that his early months with his parents had been characterised by severe neglect, which had included being locked into a cupboard. At the time of his referral when the school reported its grave concern about his hyperactivity and attentional problems, they might not have been aware that Adrian was required to have meetings with his birth mother to fulfil the statutory requirements of the Human Services Department. This was understandably an extremely stressful experience, not least because the meetings were sporadic owing to the mother's itinerant lifestyle, and it was therefore not possible to prepare Adrian properly. Adrian's foster mother described one such meeting that took place in a park. Adrian's mother arrived drunk and bore down on him like a witch in a Grimm's fairy tale to inform him that he would shortly be returning

home with her. These meetings would inevitably be followed by huge disruption in Adrian's capacity to literally 'hold himself together' to face the everyday routines of home and school.

In essence, creating links between a neuropsychological and a psychodynamic approach enables us to take a broader view of the determinants of infant and young child development and of ADHD. As McFadyen puts it, development consists of infants and young children going through a process of learning. Their parents, teachers and other caregivers need to provide the appropriate attachment contexts in which they can *learn how to use their minds* in order to regulate their mental and interpersonal functioning.

The impact of breakdown of emotional regulation

Van der Kolk (1998) asserts that the breakdown of the capacity for self-regulation, particularly in infancy and early childhood, is one of the most crucial aspects of psychological trauma. The loss or absence of self-regulation in a child interferes with their ability to think clearly about presenting stimuli and to judge what would be the best behavioural response. Van der Kolk suggests that the loss of self-regulation might be expressed at later stages of the child's development on a number of different levels. These include attentional problems, a loss of the capacity to focus on appropriate stimuli and an inability to inhibit action when aroused.

Van der Kolk confirms the importance of the style of attachment behaviour between the child and their caregivers, since unresponsive or abusive parents might promote states of chronic hyperarousal that have long-term effects on the child's capacity to modulate emotions. The child's experience of being overwhelmed by extreme emotional states might produce long-lasting alterations in physiological reactivity and affect brain development. Van der Kolk includes a variety of other traumas apart from parental abuse that can affect children in this way. These include children traumatised through accidents, repeated surgical procedures, chronic medical illness, forced separations and the witnessing of violence.

Thus we can see that the child's capacity to control emotional states in early and later childhood is dependent largely on the nature and quality of the interrelationship between the biological and the social and emotional. Rima Shore (1997) quotes a study by Megan Gunnar of the University of Minnesota, which illustrates this point. Gunnar assessed stress levels in children by measuring the amount of a hormone called cortisol in their saliva. Traumatic and adverse experiences are said to increase the level of cortisol in the human body. Higher levels of cortisol in turn affect the metabolism, the immune system and the brain. Children who have chronically high levels of cortisol through repeated traumatic events in their lives have been found to experience more developmental delays than other children (Gunnar, 1996). However, a further aspect of Gunnar's research centred on protective factors. She found that children who had received nurturing and sensitive care in their first year of life were less likely than other children to respond to minor stresses by producing cortisol and that its production in these children appeared to be more short-lived.

Some of the most compelling evidence for the pre-eminence of the attachment relationship and its vital functions of protecting the child and laying the foundations for emotional, social and cognitive development is found in longitudinal studies. Shore (1997) refers to one such study, the Minnesota Parent Child Project carried out by Egeland et al., of a long-term investigation of high-risk families since 1975. The research project started with 267 women in the last trimester of their first pregnancy, whose incomes placed them below the poverty line. Twenty years later, 180 children were still participating in the study. A variety of assessments of this group of children and parents have been carried out in order to obtain comprehensive information about the quality of each child's adaptation—social, emotional and cognitive. Over twenty years, the researchers found that infant–parent attachments at one year of age accurately predicted a child's subsequent quality of relationships in the school setting, teachers' ratings and social competency. Adverse experiences such as poverty, abuse, neglect and trauma in the early years were found to have a long-term negative cumulative effect on children's development.

The researchers also identified the factors that create resilience in children: emotionally sensitive caregiving, a well organised home environment, well developed intellectual and language capacities and a low overall level of risk. They conclude that the best way to protect children from negative trajectories is to reduce the level of stress they experience and to provide support for the family. These broader social factors bring us back to Winnicott's 'facilitating environment' and are discussed in more detail in our subsequent chapters.

Self-regulation: The point of contact between the psychodynamic and neuropsychological approaches to ADHD?

The capacity for self-regulation has been mentioned as a psychodynamic concept important in understanding ADHD, and some evidence was presented for a link between early childhood experiences and changes to brain structure and function. In fact, a number of developmental neuropsychologists have also advanced the proposition that the condition primarily represents delayed or compromised development of the brain functions responsible for the management and self-regulation of behaviour and thought, although it is not usually discussed within a psychodynamic framework. This section will present some of the current thinking with respect to this neuropsychological perspective on self-regulation and its relationship to ADHD.

While the concept of self-regulation has a history of investigation and interpretation extending back to the beginning of psychology as a scientific discipline (James, 1890) and through into the more recent cognitive-behavioural work of Kanfer (1992), Baumeister et al. (1994) and others, neuropsychologists usually discuss the construct in relation to the *executive functions*.

Self-regulation and the executive functions

The executive functions are a relatively new neuropsychological construct (Lezak, 1995; Stuss & Benson, 1984) and further empirical research is still required to tease out the full extent of their role, especially in the developing child (Anderson, 1998). They are believed to represent the individual adaptive capacities for organising the respective cognitive components necessary for completing the problems encountered in activities of daily life. Among these capacities are those that are responsible for imposing structure on a task, formulating goals and planning how to achieve them, maintaining a problem-solving set, responding to feedback and ensuring the task is completed to satisfactory standards. Lezak (1995) summarises these components as volition, planning, purposeful behaviour and effective performance.

As the main proponent of the view that the delayed development of the executive functions is the critical element in ADHD,

Barkley (1997a b & c; 1998a; 1998b) emphasises the evidence that a primary deficit in behavioural inhibition is responsible for the disorder. According to this account, deficient inhibition produces characteristic disturbances in working memory, internalisation of speech, self-regulation of emotion and the capacity for creative or flexible problem solving, all of which are part of his conceptualisation of the executive functions.

Working memory

One of the purposes of working memory is to hold information in mind for further processing. Barkley proposes that the ability to delay responding is essential for the operation of this memory system and that the contents of working memory are regularly disrupted by competing interference in children with ADHD. The failure of nonverbal working memory produced by this disruptive process results in a characteristic difficulty in imitating complex sequences, ordering events across time, utilising information from the past and developing self-awareness.

Internalisation of speech

Compromised verbal working memory in these children results in delayed internalisation of speech and consequent problems with rule-governed behaviour. The importance of the internalisation of speech as a means of self-regulation and motivation has already been mentioned with reference to the work of Luria and Vygotsky, the original proponents of the concept approximately 40 years ago. This private, self-directed speech normally develops in older primary school children to replace the audible muttering that preschoolers use to remind themselves of how to perform a task or cope with a problem. According to Barkley, the difficulty with behavioural inhibition experienced by children with ADHD is that they fail to develop this executive function and so are deprived of an important source of behavioural self-control.

Self-regulation of emotion

Working memory is necessary for the self-directed speech and visual imagery that are required for the modulation of affective states and for the capacity to sustain goal-directed behaviour. The interference in the action of working memory caused by the failure of the inhibitory processes in those with ADHD is said by Barkley to allow these children to continue to be controlled by their immediate environment rather than by internally generated states.

Behavioural analysis/reconstitution

Barkley notes that children with ADHD exhibit a diminished capacity for the behavioural analysis/reconstitution that is necessary for behavioural flexibility and efficient problem solving. By this he means that their difficulty with behavioural inhibition leads to a problem in disassembling information into units that can then be re-synthesised into novel and creative representations. One result of this is the behavioural disorganisation, rigidity and lack of creativity that is characteristic of the condition.

Evidence from a number of sources is presented by Barkley to support his proposal that ADHD is primarily manifested in deficient inhibition and impulse control. This evidence relates to problems these children experience with following instructions, delaying gratification and resisting temptation (Campbell et al., 1994). The studies that have related ADHD to increased rates of adolescent substance abuse, accidental injury/death and generally lowered life spans are also relevant here. Health psychologists have long recognised that most health compromising behaviour originates, not from lack of knowledge about the risks of actions such as smoking or speeding, but from the inability of people to put their knowledge into practice (Kaplan, Sallis & Patterson, 1993). It is significant that this discrepancy between 'knowing and doing' is accepted by many neuropsychologists as the defining characteristic of those with executive function deficit.

As indicated in Chapter 2, the executive functions have in the past most commonly been localised to the frontal lobes of the brain, and in much of the neuropsychological literature the executive functions are often described as 'frontal lobe functions'. This conceptualisation appears to be changing somewhat and other areas of the brain are increasingly being seen to be essential for the efficient performance of executive processes. Barkley, on the basis of the imaging evidence provided by Castellanos (1996) and described earlier in this book, localises those executive functions involved in ADHD to the right prefrontal cortex, to two of the basal ganglia (the caudate nucleus and the globus pallidus) and to the vermis region in the cerebellum. These structures are indicated on the diagram presented in Chapter 2.

In simple terms it can be said that the prefrontal cortex is the command centre of the brain and the caudate nucleus and globus pallidus select those commands that are to be passed on.

The net effect of Barkley's framework is to downgrade the 'inattention' of children with ADHD from a primary symptom to one that is secondary to the executive function deficits associated with disordered self-regulation. In evaluating the utility of this position it is important to remember the heterogeneity of the condition and the improbability of a single cause or explanation. This model might account for the behaviours of children who primarily have difficulties with impulsivity, but it might be inappropriate for those with specific attentional deficits. There are many studies of children diagnosed with ADHD that have not found the relationships claimed by Barkley and there are also enormous problems in establishing that executive function deficits account for these attentional problems rather than the other way around.

The complexities in the relationship between attention and the executive functions have been discussed in a number of publications but in practical terms the issue might not even be relevant. Barkley's recommendations for the way these children should be treated under this revised framework appear identical to the management approaches associated with the more traditional explanations, which focus on the child's difficulty in maintaining attention.

These recommendations are also consistent with those that follow from a psychodynamic perspective on the problem. The needs of these children for structure and 'containment' in their dealings with the world have been discussed within the context of a changing social climate. In many respects this is the point at which all of the approaches to the difficulties of these children converge. Consistency, structure and responsiveness on the part of the child's major caregivers and of the broader social ecology in which they operate might well be the keys to the operationalisation of the preventive theme running through this book.

It is also important to note that Barkley's conclusion that genetic abnormalities are probably responsible for most of the variability in the condition does not preclude a stress diathesis model, similar to that which has been proposed for schizophrenia and other conditions that present similar diagnostic dilemmas to those posed by ADHD. In this model a genetic predisposition to the condition lies

dormant until stressful environmental conditions elicit the behavioural characteristics of the syndrome. Such an account fits perfectly
with the biopsychosocial approach introduced in the next chapter,
and might well provide the theoretical framework for a final integration of the aetiological perspectives held by the psychodynamic
and neuropsychological positions.

7

ADHD in a public health context

An approach that might be more useful than the medical model in understanding the needs of children who have attentional and behavioural problems can be derived from the biopsychosocial framework (Engel, 1977, 1980; Schwartz, 1982). Such an approach moves away from an exclusive emphasis on diagnosis as a precursor to medically oriented treatment and attempts to place the condition within the context of the child's social and psychological circumstances.

Increasingly used as a framework within health psychology to better account for the majority of physical and psychiatric conditions, the biopsychosocial model is intimately related to dynamic systems theory, an analytical strategy that focuses on the fluid inter-relationships between the components of inherently changeable phenomena (Bertalanffy, 1973). The dynamic and fluctuating nature of attention is almost its defining characteristic and so, as well as being an excellent representation of the way the attention system works, systems theory is especially appropriate for considering the complexities in the aetiology and management of attentional problems. When applied through the biopsychosocial model, systems theory infers that diffuse and multidimensional conditions such as ADHD cannot be isolated or reduced to individual and specific causes but are usually the result of an intricate combination of biological, psychological and social factors that are in a constant state of reciprocal interdependence. Workers using this holistic and multifactorial approach attempt to integrate information from all three areas and to tease out the complex interactions that govern the expression of both normal and abnormal human behaviour. Rather than having as their primary focus the attachment of a diagnostic label, there is a greater concern with establishing in as much detail as possible the *context* of the problematic attentional and self-regulatory deficits.

In view of the problems that follow from an approach that is overwhelmingly dependent on accepting the applicability of the *medical model* to ADHD (see Chapter 3), the *biopsychosocial model* offers several other distinct advantages.

The biopsychosocial model is able to accept the heterogeneous aetiology of ADHD

As indicated by the evolving nomenclature that has been used to describe the disorder, there has always been a tension between the behavioural expression of ADHD (as hyperactivity–impulsivity) and its supposed aetiology in cognitive processes related to the regulation of attention. In fact there is still significant debate about the relationship between the cognitive and behavioural components of the syndrome, debate that has been fuelled by the failure to find strong correlations between the cognitive *tests* that are used by clinicians and the actual *behaviours* reported by parents and teachers (Barkley, 1992). This ongoing tension is reflected in the changing mix over time of the items that comprise the DSM diagnostic criteria for the condition. Each new revision (there have been two since the first use of the descriptive term *Attention Deficit Disorder* in 1980) has appeared to shift the emphasis among the components of the syndrome. It is interesting to note that each revision has changed the makeup of the group 'caught' by the diagnosis. For example, with the application of the latest DSM-IV there is a greater proportion of girls and preschoolers who meet the criteria compared with DSM-IIIR (Lahey et al., 1994), even though the criteria themselves are more stringent.

The heterogeneity of the items within the DSM taxonomy supports the previously discussed notion that ADHD is not a unitary diagnosis and justifies the increasing acceptance of a number of subtypes, which appear to represent conditions with variable causes and behavioural manifestations. While the medical model struggles to accommodate the idea of a single diagnosis with several aetiologies, the biopsychosocial model is flexible enough to cope with such a 'messy' conclusion and to allow an individualised interpretation of the origins of the condition for each child. Some of these contributing elements within each of the major factors are discussed in the next section.

Biological factors in ADHD

In addition to the evidence that is derived from the (albeit disputed) responsiveness of children to treatment with stimulants, a biological contribution to the aetiology of ADHD is supported by the finding of an increased risk of the condition in the parents, siblings and second-degree relatives of ADHD children. Biederman et al. (1991) found the risk in the relatives of children with ADHD was 27 per cent compared with a 5 per cent risk in the control population. Goodman and Stevenson (1989) found that about half the variance in measures of hyperactivity and inattentiveness could be accounted for by genetic effects.

This conclusion might need some qualification. While the evidence from these twin and adoption studies is often invoked to support a genetic link (Eaves et al., 1993; Faraone, 1996), the methodologies in many of the investigations have been so poor as to make the results difficult to interpret. At least one major review of the literature has concluded that there is little support for any significant genetic effect (Hinshaw, 1994) and it is still unclear whether the familial association is genetic, psychosocial, or both. More direct evidence of the link has emerged from the finding that genetic abnormalities such as Fragile X (Hagerman et al., 1992) and some congenital thyroid disorders (Weiss et al., 1993) are associated with the condition.

The contribution of biological factors is also supported by the evidence that maternal behaviours such as smoking and alcohol abuse during pregnancy appear to increase the risk of behaviours typical of ADHD in the children of these mothers (Streissguth et al., 1994). The number of studies that have found an association between attentional disorders and elevated bodily lead (e.g. Needleman et al., 1990), head injury and pre-, peri- and postnatal complications further strengthens the thesis that biology probably contributes a significant proportion of the variability in attentional ability.

Although the inability of psychophysiological measures and brain imaging techniques to reliably diagnose the condition has already been emphasised, the rapid growth in the sophistication and availability of these techniques is certain to produce further gains in our knowledge of the biology of attention. Similarly, the expanding technology of gene research might, when combined with these other findings, increase our understanding of the elements that either mark ADHD or predispose a person to develop the disorder. It is important that these findings be kept in perspective, however. For instance, it is now accepted by health psychologists that even those physical conditions that originate with genetic abnormality, viral infection or lesion are invariably influenced in their timing, presentation and impact by psychological and social factors unique to the individual.

Psychological factors in ADHD

Among the many psychological factors that have been associated with ADHD are the experience of early school failure and the degree to which the classroom and family environments are structured rather than chaotic. While these factors are known to interact with other psychological considerations, such as a demanding early temperament or an extroverted personality, there is a major problem in establishing the direction of causality. Do poor self-esteem, difficult parent–child interactions and disruptive behaviour cause the attentional disorder or are these merely outcome variables that result from the child's attempts at coping with the condition? Other individual factors that are associated with ADHD include deficient social skills; immature play behaviours and a cognitive tendency to misinterpret the intentions and behaviour of others as malicious. It is significant that all of these predisposing attributes are amenable to intervention.

Social factors in ADHD

There is no doubt that changing social conditions have influenced the extent to which disturbances in attention and behaviour have been observed in children. The effects of busier lifestyles, increased levels of family breakdown and rapidly changing structures within society were fully discussed in Chapter 4. In this section we focus on the social factors within the biopsychosocial model that have been clearly identified by epidemiological research as influencing the diagnosis and treatment of the condition.

The sway held by social factors in the diagnosis and treatment of ADHD is most clearly observed in the gender differences in incidence rates between clinic and community samples. In those actually referred for assessment, the ratio is about six males to every one female (Barkley, 1990). In community-based samples, however, where the children being examined are not only those for whom help is being sought, the ratio comes down to somewhere between three to one (Szatmari, Offord & Boyle, 1989) and two to one (Sawyer et al., 2000), a reduction that appears to indicate that gender expectations are very important in determining referral and hence diagnosis. The expression of the disorder in boys appears to be much more disruptive to parents and teachers, while for girls more severe behaviours must be displayed before a referral is made. Girls are therefore often older than boys at the time of referral (Brown et al., 1991). This evidence supports the previously introduced finding that the social settings in which the behaviours occur largely determine whether they come to be considered the 'symptoms' of an underlying 'medical' condition such as ADHD. There are many studies within the medical sociology literature that have come to similar conclusions regarding the cultural determinants of 'conditions' such as menstrual pain, obesity, headache and back injury (Delaney, Lupton & Toth, 1988; Helman, 1984; Whitehead et al., 1986).

Socioeconomic status is another factor that needs to be entered into the complex equation necessary to describe the prevalence and aetiology of the condition. While the bias in the assessment process discussed in Chapter 2 might inflate the differential tendency for children from lower socioeconomic strata to receive the diagnosis, there are increasing reports of a real variability in the incidence rate of the condition across the classes (Denckla, 1991; Prosser, 1999). Reflecting the complex nature of the interaction, however, is the evidence that the effect of socioeconomic status might be bidirectional as well as influenced by other mediating variables. Barkley (1990), for example, refers to the downward 'social drift' experienced by individuals with the disorder. This drift is hypothesised to result from a number of factors, including the lowered benefits from education derived by this group and the evidence for the hereditability of the condition. The differential incidence of stress across the socioeconomic groups, together with a lower utilisation of mental health and prenatal services in lower-class children, might also account for some of this variability (Helman, 1984; Sanson, Smart, Prior & Oberklaid, 1993).

Further evidence of the contribution of social factors to ADHD comes from the already noted finding that they are a major determinant of outcome following intervention. Chief among these social factors is the family's socioeconomic status. In children diagnosed with ADHD, as with undiagnosed children, the extent of the financial resources available to the family is the most important predictor of the child's level of academic achievement and later work success (Barkley, 1998a).

The real strength of the biopsychosocial model lies in its capacity to integrate the elements contributing to a diverse syndrome such as ADHD, and to describe the complex interactions among them that eventually determine the decision to attach the psychiatric label. For example, it is easy to imagine a child with a slight biological vulnerability within a chaotic and economically disadvantaged home environment exhibiting all of the classic problematic behaviours that comprise the DSM diagnostic criteria. In this case the nature of the family's circumstances would predict a negative interaction between these elements, leading to an unfavourable outcome. It is just as easy to imagine how the same child with one or more of these elements absent or moderated by the influence of other more positive factors might never even come into consideration for being 'at risk'. Systems theory acknowledges that small variations within the components that contribute to complex and multidetermined phenomena might have significant multiplier effects that are inherent in the interdependent relationships that exist between those elements. The example that is most frequently cited to explain these interactions is the so-called 'butterfly effect' in which the beating of a butterfly's wings in the Amazon can result in a cyclone off the coast of Indonesia. The medical model, relying as it does on the identification and description of relationships that are essentially linear and additive in nature, is incapable of accounting for this level of complexity, yet the analysis of multifactorial behavioural conditions such as ADHD demands it.

The propensity for humans to search for unitary explanatory causes for behavioural disturbances has been extensively investigated and might account for some of the biomedical bias in the conceptualisation of ADHD (Nisbett & Ross, 1980). Such single cause–effect models also have some reinforcing advantages in saving us from information overload and saving on cost when clinician time and energy are the main costs considered.

The biopsychosocial model rejects the pathological–normal dichotomy

The biopsychosocial model accepts that ADHD's identifying cluster of 'symptoms' is simply an exaggerated presentation of normal behaviours. They are not unique in themselves and it is impossible to draw a distinct line between their normal and their pathological expression, except in a limited statistical sense. These behavioural tendencies are neither inherently pathological nor intrinsically dysfunctional and many adults and children with the condition might find some of the behaviours advantageous in certain circumstances. The literature on residual ADHD in adults is replete with case studies of individuals who have adjusted to the negative elements of the diagnosis and who have been able therefore to exploit the more positive aspects associated with above-average levels of energy, drive and desire for stimulation. Occupational choice is obviously an important consideration here, reflecting the high degree of situational specificity of ADHD symptoms. One study that followed up ADHD children into adulthood found that 18 per cent owned small businesses compared with only 5 per cent of controls. The authors speculated that one reason for this imbalance was the high level of activity and willingness to take entrepreneurial risks associated with the condition (Mannuzza et al., 1993).

The biopsychosocial model accepts the need for multidisciplinary intervention

The biopsychosocial model advocates the need for a number of disciplines to be involved in the planning and implementation of interventions. The heterogeneous nature of the syndrome means that no one discipline can claim complete expertise. The adoption of an approach derived from systems theory means that a simple suggestion or procedure originating from one of the many disciplinary perspectives on the condition might produce quite dramatic interactional effects in the context of the other approaches being applied.

This is not to suggest that disproven therapies should be persisted with in the hope that some flukish combination with more orthodox strategies might produce a 'cure'. This is especially so since the biopsychosocial model moves away from an emphasis on finding a cure to the goal of reaching a state where the interaction of biological, psychological and social factors achieves a condition sufficiently stable as to minimise disruptive effects.

It is useful here to identify those treatments that have been found to be ineffective and those found to be effective. Evaluations of these approaches have been presented in the reviews conducted by the National Health and Medical Research Council in Australia (1997), the National Institute of Health in America (1998), the Ministry of Health in New Zealand (2001) and the British Psychological Society (1996). The approaches that have been found *not* to be effective in any general sense include:

- eye training/coloured lens
- chiropractic adjustment
- restrictive diet/megavitamins
- allergy treatments.

Consistent with the framework offered by the biopsychosocial model, research suggests that the more effective interventions typically operate across family and school boundaries and are not simply focused on the child presenting the 'symptoms'. Family-based interventions appear to be more successful than those directed at the child as a passive *patient*. Among the approaches that have been found to achieve some degree of positive outcome are:

- support groups/parenting skills training
- social skills training/family therapy
- cognitive behaviour therapy
- psychotherapy.

An emphasis on a public health approach

The biopsychosocial model accepts a proactive, preventive approach to problems with attention and impulse control. A move away from the medical model allows for the development of a much broader based set of proactive interventions. Rather than remaining firmly fixed on the necessity for individual diagnosis as a precursor to treatment, the focus changes to a set of objectives that may be likened to those espoused by the public health movement. The medical model's concern with the individual is replaced with a more efficient population emphasis; and the search for a *cure* is replaced with a more realistic determination to make environmental or social modifications that have the capacity to lower the incidence of the condition within the community or to minimise the appearance of *symptoms*. Concomitant with this change in emphasis, the medical model's focus on the reactive treatment of the individual's pathology is replaced with the goal of enhancing health and wellbeing in the community using proactive policy decisions. In the case of ADHD many of the prescriptive recommendations, which are often made for 'managing' the behaviour of the relatively small number of children who can be unequivocally diagnosed with the disorder, are able to be translated into broad suggestions that are useful in a preventive and health promoting sense for *all* children—whether or not they have received a diagnostic label. This was also the conclusion reached by the ADHD working party of the British Psychological Society (1996) who noted that 'intervention strategies recommended under the heading of ADHD are also beneficial for other children because effective parenting and teaching takes account of individual differences and tailors interactions and environmental demands accordingly' (p. 7).

In fact the utility of the public health approach to the problems associated with attention disorders in children is especially appropriate because these conditions represent a significant public health risk in themselves. Research suggests that children with ADHD exhibit higher rates of accidental injuries through misadventure (Pless, Taylor & Arsenault, 1995) and that when they reach adolescence they become more susceptible to substance abuse (Ahadpour, Horton & Vaeth, 1993), depression and suicide (Weiss & Hechtman, 1993). At this period in their lives they are three times more likely to be involved in car accidents than are adolescents who have not received the diagnosis (Pless, Taylor & Arsenault, 1995), and they are five times more likely to become caught up in the criminal justice system (Eyestone & Howell, 1994; Forehand et al., 1991). These studies, together with the evidence for increased prevalence of other health-risking behaviours such as smoking, caffeinism, teenage pregnancy and poor diet (Milberger et al., 1996), justify the conclusion that the condition significantly reduces life expectancy (Barkley, 1997a) and exacts a huge economic and social toll on the community[1]. In public health terminology these costs are referred to as the *burden* of the disease.

A first stage in a typical public health campaign is an epidemiological analysis of the extent of the problem. In the case of ADHD the difficulties associated with estimating the incidence of the condition have already been described. Although most assessments are that less than 5 per cent of children have 'pure' ADHD, the number of children experiencing attentional difficulties with alternative aetiologies is likely to be far higher, possibly running into billions of people the world over (Mirsky, 1995). An epidemiological study of an urban population in Chicago found 15–25 per cent of first-graders with moderate to severe concentration problems (Kellam, Branch, Agrawal & Ensminger, 1975). In the Isle of Wight study in the UK (Rutter, Tizard & Whitmore, 1970), 30 per cent of an epidemiological population of schoolchildren experienced attentional problems.

At the school level it can confidently be asserted that within any one classroom many children would have experienced one or more of the many risk factors associated with attention deficits. These include encephalitis, meningitis, epilepsy, autism, Tourette's syndrome, chronic ear infections, exposure to lead from paint or petrol exhausts, treatments for medical conditions such as leukaemia or epilepsy, head injuries resulting from falls and motor vehicle accidents, anxiety, depression, learning disorder and developmental delay.

The classroom incidence of attention disorders is likely to be higher in school districts with active mainstreaming programs or in areas of socioeconomic deprivation. The risk factors for attentional problems that have been directly associated with poverty include foetal exposure to alcohol, exposure to lead, malnutrition, neurocysticerosis (a parasitic infection of the brain) and cultural impoverishment (Mirsky, 1995).

Obviously the most effective public health response to this situation is to attempt to prevent these risk factors from occurring in the first place—in the same way that John Snow famously dealt with the London cholera epidemic of the 1850s by disabling the pump of the infected water supply. As well as the obvious financial constraint on this strategy when applied to the wide range of risk factors for attentional problems, one reason why authorities have been relatively tardy in following this approach is that knowledge about the subtle effects of these events on the information processing capacities of children is only just emerging. In the case of head injuries, for example, it has always been believed that the brains of young children (compared with those of adults) were relatively 'plastic', even in the face of severe trauma. One element in the reasoning behind this conclusion was evidence that young children appeared to be capable of remarkable recoveries from operations in which a large amount of brain tissue was removed. The apparent ability of other areas of the brain to take over the function of the excised tissue has been termed 'neuronal plasticity'; however, it is only now becoming clear that these processes are not as effective in producing complete recovery as was first thought. Recent research indicates that even minor head injuries received when children are very young place them at significant risk for the later development of attentional problems that have the capacity to impact upon school success and behaviour (Anderson & Pentland, 1998; Catroppa, Anderson & Stargatt, 1999). Growing awareness of this newly uncovered risk factor has already resulted in mandatory bicycle helmet and child restraint legislation in many countries. Local councils are becoming more selective in playground design and national health and safety organisations are increasingly active in urging the removal of commercial products associated with risk of head injury in young children. The campaign to inform the public of the dangers of baby-walkers is an example of this increased awareness. In a similar fashion the increased knowledge of the effects of lead on attentional abilities has resulted in the lowering of lead levels in petrol, the replacement of leaded petrol with AVGAS in Aboriginal communities, the complete banning of lead-based paints and the replacement of the lead solder previously used in canning processes with spot-welding techniques.

The social ecology of the classroom

A less obvious public health approach to reducing the community incidence of attention disorder focuses on those *social* environments where the behavioural manifestations of attentional difficulties are likely to be expressed. In many cases these will be school classrooms. One study has found, for example, that some classroom milieus, labelled 'provocation ecologies', tend to accentuate the attentional problems of children whereas other environments, referred to as 'rarification ecologies', appear to ameliorate the same difficulties. Provocation ecologies are those in which the discipline structure within the classroom is either unusually rigid or completely absent, and where noise is either tolerated to a distracting degree or completely forbidden. By way of contrast, teachers in rarification ecologies are flexible in their reactions to minor disruptions but provide sufficient structure so that children know what they should be doing and when they should be doing it (Whalen et al., 1979).

The reasons for the differential effects of these classroom environments can be clearly understood in the light of current knowledge of the behavioural and cognitive expression of attentional deficits in children. For example, in the case where a child has trouble with focusing attention, it is the filtering mechanism that is not coping with environmental demands. Extraneous stimulation from distracting images and background noise appears to overload the child's capacity to successfully deal with the incoming data. The difficulties encountered in filtering out irrelevant input might result irr inefficient processing of the teacher's instructions and possibly an inability to carry them out. Quieter environments, such as those provided in the rarification ecologies, act to minimise the strain placed on these mechanisms while still allowing enough stimulation to maintain adequate levels of arousal.

In the case of children with deficits in executive functioning, the imposed structure provided by classroom routine can compensate for difficulties experienced in supervising the allocation of attentional resources. Where the majority of organisational decisions have already been made for the child, processing resources can be freed up for allocation to a much smaller number of chosen or assigned tasks. There is also less potential for children to use their limited attentional capacity attending to irrelevant, non-task-related stimuli.

Research has also demonstrated that the protective effect of rarification ecologies can be enhanced if teachers:

- make the classroom routine explicit by discussing the day's events and expectations first thing in the morning to prepare children and avoid potential problems;
- present logically organised lessons that are carefully pitched at the child's level of ability so as to prevent the overburdening of children's processing resources;
- clearly describe the links between new material and prior knowledge;
- assist children with setting work priorities by structuring and sequencing larger assignments and tasks for the students to prevent them from becoming overwhelmed.

The fluctuating performance levels of children with attentional problems have already been commented on with reference to the unreliability of conventional diagnostic procedures with this group of children. This performance variability is known to occur over both short and long intervals, although much of the clinical research has focused on the abnormally large decrease in performance between morning and afternoon periods. As indicated in Chapter 2, the capacity to maintain attention is essentially the responsibility of the brain-stem reticular activating system, a mechanism that is subject to daily changes associated with the circadian rhythm. A preventive public health approach to minimising the symptoms of attention deficits would promote the structuring of the classroom environment so that the acknowledged higher levels of arousal in morning periods were exploited for the completion of difficult or low-interest work. This is an obvious facilitative policy that has been adopted by generations of teachers as appropriate for the learning of all students, not just those with attentional problems.

Changes to other elements of the child's physical environment that can assist in the prevention of attentional problems relate to classroom design issues. The trend to large 'open-plan' learning areas in schools that began in the 1970s has exerted a toll on the capacity of children with marginal attentional resources to focus on the relevant material and exclude the irrelevant. New school designs should reflect increasing knowledge of the limitations of many children in effectively performing this attention allocation function.

The actual teaching strategies adopted by educators represent an important aspect of the child's environment that might be manipulated to meet the public health objective of limiting the incidence of attention disorder. We referred earlier to the concept of verbal mediation based on the ideas of Vygotsky (1962) and his student Luria (1961), two influential Russian neuropsychologists who proposed that the regulation of attention is largely dependent on *subvocal* or *inner speech*. Luria (1961) described three stages in the development of self-regulation in children: a) the speech of others controls and directs the child's behaviour; b) the child's own overt speech begins to control their behaviour; c) the content/meaning of the child's covert speech effectively regulates their behaviour. He proposed that the self-regulation of this inner speech could intervene when behaviour problems were due to neural processes that were immature, damaged or dysfunctional and demonstrated these verbal-mediation techniques with children with a syndrome similar to hyperactivity. These ideas have been adapted to a number of cognitive–behavioural programs specifically developed for use with children presenting with attentional problems (Sohlberg & Mateer, 2001).

While a reversion to the traditional 'chalk and talk' teaching style—previously made necessary in the 1940s and 1950s by large class sizes—would be catastrophic for students with marginal attentional resources, these children do respond well to a teaching style known as 'direct instruction' (Kameenui & Simmons, 1990). The direct instruction model of curriculum design was developed by Engelmann and Carnine (1982). It involves explicit, highly structured, one-to-one teaching, which includes the identification of what is to be taught and why, the demonstration of each micro-skill by the teacher and the engagement of the student in guided practice with immediate feedback. Skills are individually identified and reinforced using verbal mediation techniques where the teacher simultaneously demonstrates and verbally describes a task or thought process. The child is then asked to repeat the steps of the problem as they work through it and the teacher provides immediate corrective feedback.

The social ecology of the family

The social ecology within families is another point of leverage where public health policies might act to alter environments that have been demonstrated to increase risk. For example, maternal depression is consistently implicated as a risk factor for ADHD in children, although Rutter (1990) suggests that rather than there being a direct relationship, the mediating factor is the negative interactional styles that are set up in these circumstances. Whatever the relationship, it is clear that recent government initiatives directed at countering the epidemic of depression in the community will have an enormous long-term effect in improving family relationships even though they are not specifically directed at parent support.

Writers such as Belsky (1984) and Bronfenbrenner (1986) have developed a theoretical framework around the family ecology model, often extending their discussion to take into account the wider social context such as social policy, cultural belief systems and unemployment. Unfortunately, the increased recognition of the effectiveness of parenting and parent support programs in reducing the risk of conduct disorder has coincided with a period in which direct access to government-funded psychological services for families is being rationed to an extent not seen in many years. As well as decreasing the availability of these proactive family intervention programs, reduced levels of service have had the countereffect of increasing the reliance on reactive and shortcut approaches to complex behaviour problems. The explosion in prescription rates for dexamphetamine/methylphenidate and the common use of these psychostimulants as diagnostic challenges by paediatricians under pressure can be seen as representing the most visible outcome of these funding reductions.

Another area of government policy that has been instrumental in increasing the population incidence of ADHD is the current emphasis on a medical diagnosis as supporting evidence for integration assistance in schools. Parents are forced into a practice akin to 'doctor shopping' for a medical or psychiatric label so that their child can gain access to support. In contrast, the biopsychosocial model anticipates the dependence of behavioural states on situational and social factors that may fluctuate and change rapidly. An important implication that flows from an acceptance of the biopsychosocial model is the undesirability of applying something as permanent as a psychiatric label to a child for the achievement of goals that might be more effectively met using contextual strategies. Government policy should not encourage people to see themselves as 'victims' of their own biology.

Reid, Maag and Vasa (1994) have argued persuasively against proposals by various advocacy groups to make ADHD a separate educational disability category. These proposals have originated in response to the increasing difficulty schools are experiencing in meeting the demands of parents for support for their children out of existing school funding. Reid et al. argue that the diagnosis is ultimately irrelevant to the educational needs of children, except for providing access to medication. They say that in some cases labelling a child's difficulties with a medical tag can actually be counterproductive to the provision of appropriate special education services because teachers often relinquish responsibility for the child once medical issues become involved.

It is important to remember that while problems with attention might persist with varying symptomatology into adulthood (Denckla, 1991), the dysfunctional consequences of these disturbances tend to diminish over time as the brain reaches maturity and coping strategies are developed (Hechtman, 1991). Research has consistently demonstrated that the most significant predictors of long-term outcome are the socioeconomic status of the family, the intelligence level of the child, the extent of the conduct/relationship problems experienced and the mental health of the child's parents.

The factors that appear to be most protective against poor outcome include the availability of supportive and empowered adults who are prepared to advocate for the child, the presence of a strong parental coalition with satisfactory child management skills and the availability of effective community resources. Thus the predominantly psychosocial nature of these predictors provides further compelling evidence that conceptualising ADHD purely in terms of the medical model provides a grossly inadequate account of the nature of the 'condition', its likely course and the most effective forms of intervention.

8

Coming full circle: Towards a new paradigm for helping children, parents and families

In chapters 1 and 7 we referred to the need for a new paradigm that can assist us to make sense of attentional problems in children and young people. We made the point that an essential part of any paradigm shift in this area involves a move away from an individual pathology-based medical model to one that encompasses the broader child and family public mental health domain.

In this chapter we outline first what we consider to be a more appropriate conceptual and theoretical framework for understanding the nature of attentional problems. Second we describe how the services that are offered to children, parents and families themselves need to undergo a fundamental paradigm shift if these problems are to be addressed effectively.

The need for a new paradigm

The theme throughout this book is that ADHD viewed as 'an illness for our time' suggests that the problem is in fact the tip of the iceberg of multi-factorial behaviours whose aetiology resides in the complex interrelationship between individual social and emotional experience as well as broader family, economic and cultural factors.

Such a view enables us to assume that all behaviour has meaning. Understanding the problem of the child diagnosed with ADHD inevitably leads us to an understanding of *all* children. It follows therefore that any recommendations made for this group of children are relevant to the development and emotional growth of *all* children.

Reviewing basic assumptions

As we have stated from the outset, while the complexity of attentional problems calls for greater synthesis, integration and communication between disciplines, the reality is often a fragmented approach with different disciplines competing for *supremacy of definition*. This has led to a dangerous split in which brain function is identified as a concrete entity separate from the development of emotional and social relationships. This flies in the face of evidence from current research in neuroscience, which emphasises that for the infant and young child 'early interactions don't just create a context, they directly affect the way the brain is "wired" ' (Shore, 1997).

The need to simplify and create concrete constructs that fragment behaviour and strip it of meaning resonates with the idea that we can achieve liberation through technical knowledge. As the philosopher John Gray (1999) states, 'late modern cultures are haunted by the dream that new technologies (which include the use of chemicals to alter mood or behaviour) will conjure away the immemorial evils of human life'. In Chapter 3 we referred to the British Government's enquiry into prescriptions of psychostimulants for all school-aged children meeting the diagnostic criteria for severe combined type ADHD. The thinking behind such a potentially huge initiative is a good example of Gray's 'dream of new technologies'.

Apart from the human rights issues involved in such a proposal, it has been rightly placed in context by the director of Young Minds, the child mental health consortium in the UK (Wilson, 2000), who states that decades of underinvestment in child and adolescent mental health services have made services so overstretched that they would be unable to cope, even if all children suffering from severe ADHD were given a trial prescription of medication.

The rise in social and emotional problems

Paul Cooper (1998), writing about developments and changes in the understanding of children's emotional and behavioural problems, concurs with the findings of Rutter and Smith (1995). This is that the evidence of 50 years of social research indicates that in most countries of the developed world, things have got worse for people in relation to a wide range of psychosocial problems. Cooper further points out that one of the most consistent and reliable research findings is that adult criminality almost always follows a developmental path that begins with childhood delinquency or conduct disorder (Smith, 1995). The increased rates of psychosocial problems of all types suggest that life has become increasingly difficult for children and young people in Western society. The scope of these problems suggests that professionals can no more take total responsibility for finding solutions or treatments than they can gather the grains of sand on the beach. In other words, if we adhere to traditional problem-based pathology–treatment models, the size of the problem will always outweigh the professional resources available. Financial imperatives and constraints clearly contribute to the way in which the problem is defined. They are part of the broader social context.

Paradigm shifts

In line with our focus on a public health approach, we believe that there is a need for a change in many of the basic assumptions we make about child and family problems. We advocate the following paradigm shifts as necessary for the development of child and family mental health, of which ADHD is only one element. These paradigm shifts can be summarised as follows:

- a paradigm shift of definition;
- a paradigm shift of shared responsibility with parents;
- a paradigm shift of recognising what children can contribute.

A paradigm shift of definition: From pathology and illness to child and family wellness

A paradigm shift of definition moves us away from the narrowly focused debate about a problem *within* the child towards a conceptual framework that acknowledges the child in relation to significant interpersonal relationships and the wider community. The concept of *child and family wellness* is seen as a particular example of this shift of definition. Wellness is described as a 'favourable state of affairs, brought about by the combined presence of cogent values, satisfactory psychological and material resources, effective policies and successful programs. Basically family wellness is a state of affairs in which everybody's needs in the family are met' (Nelson & Peirson, 2001, p. 8).

Wellness is viewed as being *ecological* in nature, in that there are key interrelationships between the child, parent and family and community and wider society. This is echoed in Chapter 4 where we identify some of the risk factors for children and parents who live in a changing society that give rise to problems of attention and self-regulation.

The concept of wellness has become a cornerstone of the Canadian Early Years Study (Mustard, 1999). This innovative project was commissioned by the government of Ontario and makes the point that while parents and families have a primary role in supporting and nurturing children, they cannot carry out this task without the support and commitment of the community and wider society. Thus government businesses, non-profit organisations and professional networks all have a role to play in contributing to the wellbeing of children.

The Early Years Study confirms that new knowledge about brain development has created an even greater imperative to support development in infancy and early childhood. 'It is clear that the early years from conception to age six have the most important influence of any time in the life cycle on brain development and subsequent learning behaviour and health.' (Mustard, 1999, p. 7)

It is significant that the Early Years Study does not stop at identifying the needs of infants and young children but draws attention to the fact that positive development for young children is severely impeded by the stress experienced by families in the current climate of economic and social change. As the report states:

> our future depends on our ability to manage the complex interplay of the emerging new economy, changing social environments and the impact of change on individuals, particularly those who are most vulnerable in their formative early years—our children . . . A key strategy for improving the capabilities for innovation of the next generation of citizens is to make early child development a priority of the public and private sectors of society. (Mustard, 1999, p. 8)

A paradigm shift of shared responsibility: The involvement of parents

The current debate about the nature of ADHD is typical of many of its kind concerning psychological problems, in that it takes place primarily within the professional community. The recipients or consumers of the services—the children, adolescents and parents—take little or no part in this debate. This means that definitions of behaviour and decision making about behaviour are the domain of a minority of people—that is professionals who possess 'special knowledge'. It is a position that over the longer term encourages not only dependence, but a belief that the professional has the power and therefore should provide the answer to any problem, for example when parents expect an ADHD diagnosis 'on demand'. The medicalisation of the problem additionally serves to further shift responsibility away from parents since, as we stated earlier, it isolates the problem firmly within the child as a disease entity.

A paradigm shift of shared responsibility involves the instatement of parents as having the capacity and competence to observe and understand their own children, and to take appropriate action where necessary. An essential part of this paradigm shift is the sharing of knowledge and understanding about child development. What is generally regarded as *specialised knowledge* needs to become *common knowledge*. Another way of looking at this is to consider, for example, that we often only become aware of the importance of relationships and the dynamics of family relationships when they break down. Typically most people experience this at the point at which they seek counselling or support with a problem.

Changing the paradigm to a shared partnership between parents and professionals enables a vital component of prevention to be put in place—the capacity to be proactive literally at the source. As the Early Years Study states:

> the evidence is clear that good early child development programs that involve parents or other primary care givers of young children can influence how they relate to and care for children in the home, and can vastly improve outcomes for children's behaviour, learning and health in later life. (Mustard, 1999, p. 7)

An example of a successful parent–professional partnership model in the UK was devised by Ruth Schmidt Neven (1994) who was the founder and co-director with Carolyn Douglas of the organisation Exploring Parenthood. Exploring Parenthood was one of several pioneering organisations in parent support in the UK, which foreshadowed the current British Government's recent establishment of a National Family and Parenting Institute.

Exploring Parenthood was founded on the assumption that parents and professionals can work together to support children by sharing knowledge and information through group meetings and workshops. The aim of these group workshops is to facilitate parents' *own knowledge and understanding;* to help them to *own what they know* and literally to *find their own voice.* It is the antithesis of offering strategies and prescriptions for behaviour, which contributes to the cycle of dependence and suggests that one group, namely the professionals, has both 'the syllabus' for parenting as well as the 'answers'.

The community development focus of the organisation means that parents can become 'key contacts' in their local areas and undertake training through the organisation to develop the skills to run their own support groups. The ultimate outcome is a *community of parents* utilising a core developmental approach to parenthood that can be applied to all parents and all children in whatever situation they find themselves, rather than identifying and pathologising one particular group. A key feature of the Exploring Parenthood model is a training program in which parents and professionals learn alongside each other, thus acknowledging the skills of life experience as well as learned experience.

As the British family therapist Robin Skynner (1996) explains:

> Unlike most organizations then existing, this program (Exploring Parenthood) was based on the idea of partnership between parents and professionals, on health rather than on pathology, on prevention rather than cure, on competence rather than failure. Parents would have direct access to it, when they wished to come, rather than through professionals when some serious problems had provided an admission ticket. (p. 65).

A paradigm shift of recognising what children themselves can contribute

Much of the discourse associated with ADHD concerns itself with innumerable descriptions from professionals *about* the child or adolescent but we have very little information or contribution from children and adolescents themselves. A paradigm shift of shared responsibility implies that their voices need to be heard and their experiences and views perceived as valid.

The idea that children can actually be involved constructively in understanding their problem and in contributing to decision making about the help that might really suit them is an essential part of this paradigm shift.

This recognition is also an important element of the therapeutic process. However, here we argue that taking children and their communications seriously is a critical part of developing individual and social wellness, as defined earlier, and must necessarily go beyond the therapeutic encounter. In other words, listening to children and respecting their views and contributions not only models the basis of a civil society but also has the potential to make a contribution to preventive mental health.

It is worth noting in this regard that the United Nations Convention on the Rights of the Child foreshadows this requirement by confirming the child's right to information, to express a view and to be heard.

The UK-based organisation Save the Children has devised a number of training initiatives that assist professionals to consult children directly on issues of concern to them. Most recently this has involved talking to children about, among other things, their views on physical punishment in the home and at school. Fajerman, Jarrett and Sutton (2000) describe the approach of Save the Children, which seeks to influence policy and practice to achieve lasting benefits for children within its communities and to make children's rights a reality.

As Fajerman et al. explain, everyone benefits from the process of shared consultation; children, young people, their parents and the staff who are responsible for children in early childhood settings, schools and other community settings.

The benefits to the child are reflected in greater self-esteem, and a sense of being listened to with respect. This in turn leads to improvements in the child's capacity for independent creative learning. Interestingly, as the authors point out, it also helps to decrease conflict: 'The opportunity [for children] to express their views and negotiate reduces the potential of conflict between children and staff and children and children.' (p. 8)

The benefit for staff is that working in partnership with children enables them to facilitate and support the child's development. This also promotes improved teamwork among staff and an increased awareness of children's needs.

For parents, the benefit of working in partnership with staff is that they can obtain constant feedback from staff and from the children themselves. This is a far cry from the common dilemma in early childhood centres where staff might be too frightened to tell parents that their child has a problem, or alternatively make the problem the central focus of any discussion.

Through the partnership with staff, parents gain greater aware-ness of how children participate and learn in the group. They are also made aware of how the setting values children and their contributions.

Paradigm shifts and community health

In Chapter 7 our discussion of a public health approach referred to the famous example of John Snow, who dealt with the London cholera epidemic of the 1850s by disabling the pump of the infected water supply. This was an apt example in that improved sanitation and hygiene had more far-reaching effects on our lives and health than advances in medicine.

Public health and hygiene have been part of very successful educational initiatives, and there is every reason to believe that education and support programs could achieve similar results in supporting family and community emotional relationships. However, the key factor, as we describe above, is an acknowledge-ment and understanding of a *process* of change. This process of change must come from the development of new partnerships between professionals and families and from a recognition that there cannot be effective change unless there is as sense of owner-ship and participation in this process.

This model of developing the wellness of communities is dependent, according to community psychologist Kenneth Maton (2000), on articulating a strategic vision of social transformation. Maton proposes four of what he calls 'foundational goals' for the work of social transformation. These are:

- capacity building
- group empowerment
- relational community-building
- culture challenge.

Maton emphasises that these goals can only be achieved through a cooperative multidisciplinary, multi-agency and partnership approach, which must also involve the relevant stakeholders, namely children, parents and families. Maton emphasises the role of positive personal and intergroup relationships in contributing to a sense of individual and social wellbeing, and the ways in which this can be undermined. He cites as an example the way in which professionals construct and describe children's problems. As Maton explains, the predominant medical definitions of children's behaviour as discrete problems create a model of *deficit*. What is needed is to create a model of *wellness*, that takes as its starting point an understanding of how healthy development occurs and how children can be made resilient. This is a model that by contrast emphasises positive potential rather than deficit within the individual and draws on the strengths and competencies of the child and family. It resonates with Siegel's (2001) idea of 'a collaborative environment of nurturing communities'.

Maton's vision of social transformation, which includes interventions on multiple levels from the individual to the societal, echoes the points we have made in Chapter 4 in describing the individual and social risk factors for children. However, Maton's vision goes further in suggesting that preventive mental health for children could be greatly enhanced by the creation of a 'children's movement'. This is a movement, he says, 'in which the majority of citizens finally realise that the development of *all* children really matters, and that all children are 'our children' (p. 47).

9

Recommendations for a multidisciplinary approach to ADHD

The point has been made throughout this book that many of the behavioural difficulties of young children, particularly boys, are related to profound changes in socioeconomic structures in society, which have an influence on individual and family development. This means that there cannot be a purely clinical or medical answer to the problem. We therefore recognise the value of a broad multidisciplinary approach to helping children and families cope better with behavioural and emotional difficulties.

The recommendations we make in this chapter are both a distillation of research and understanding and a way of putting into practice the multidisciplinary proactive and preventive theme of this book.

Avoiding a disposal diagnosis

It is important for all professionals involved with children and young people to recognise that ADHD should not be used as the diagnosis of disposal for behaviour that appears to be too difficult to tolerate or manage. The danger here is that a diagnosis of ADHD can be used to cover a wide range of behaviours that have a variety of different causations. Thus, rather than looking to fit the child to the diagnosis, we need to understand the real needs of each individual child and each individual family situation.

Recognising that medication is not a cure

Even for those children for whom medication is an appropriate form of treatment, it nevertheless cannot be viewed as the sole form of treatment. Medication is best combined with other forms of help for the child, which reflect the child's overall needs as well as help for the family.

Not colluding against the child

It is important for professionals not to collude with parents in *blaming* the child for having the problem. Parents understandably might wish to deny the complexities of the difficulties they face as a family. The scapegoating of one member of the family who can be relied on to contain all the family problems is not unusual. If we take a family systems view of such a family, it becomes clear that the inattentive or overactive behaviour of a child might have a particular *function* for the family. Thus we need to understand the *meaning* of the child's behaviour in the context of the family difficulties.

Containing anxiety

It is tempting for us as professionals to believe that we can provide an answer to complex behavioural problems, and many 'spot diagnoses' of ADD or ADHD in the child might be made with the best of intentions, in the hope of alleviating stress in the parent. However, we would suggest that the task for clinicians is not to provide answers for parents but rather to assist them to *tolerate uncertainty and to contain anxiety*, so that they can find their own solutions to problems. This requires of course that professionals have access to containment for themselves in the form of regular and supportive supervision and consultation.

Expanding our understanding of the meaning of children's behaviour

Children are able to communicate a great deal about how they think and feel. Taking children seriously and being prepared to listen to them can provide a framework for prevention, whether in the family home or at school. The recent publicity in the UK and Australia surrounding the problem of bullying highlights how many children can feel and how little they might trust ↑ understand their predicament. We need to encourage greater awareness in the community of how children really behave and of the greater importance of their emotional needs relative to their material needs.

One aspect of this involves recognition of the important emotional differences between boys and girls, and the way in which boys communicate their need for intimacy. The more boisterous behaviour of boys might be misconstrued as aggression when it might in fact represent a wish to be close to a parent or teacher. The rejection of the boy's overture might lead to his becoming even more disruptive.

The need for appropriate authority and the use of boundaries

As parents and professionals we need to be clearer about the place of good authority and the importance of setting limits and offering containment to children and young people. This is the opposite of being authoritarian. Most children find unstructured environments difficult to operate in, particularly where the rules are either absent or inconsistent. A fear of saying no, of setting limits and using good authority might lead to many of the problems associated with out-of-control behaviour, since it might be construed as not caring.

Working in partnership with parents

Partnerships between parents and professionals, whether in a school setting, social work setting, therapeutic setting or childcare setting, offer ideal opportunities for the containment for children. Many professionals deplore the cuts in health and community services, but hopefully they might open up the potential for a different way of working and a different kind of enquiry. It might become quite unrealistic in the longer term for the experts and professionals to believe that they must undertake all the work by themselves, even with the best of financial resources.

If we take the view that our task as professionals is to help parents and families find their own answers and to empower their decision making then we need to institute greater opportunities for a true partnership between parents and professionals.

Parenting and prevention

On a preventive level we need to involve parents more actively, not only to understand the needs of children with attentional deficits but also to obtain more information about the developmental needs of children generally. As we have said earlier, *specialised knowledge needs to become common knowledge* so that, for example, the problem of ADHD is seen within the broader context of public health and education.

The introduction of more formalised support services for parents in Australia and overseas is a step in the right direction. However, it is often difficult for these programs to free themselves from a focus on providing strategies and quick-fix solutions for dealing with children's problems rather than on helping parents to learn how *to process* the complexity of family events and make connections.

There is also a need to redress the current imbalance in many parent education programs in which there is a strong focus on the needs and requests of parents, with less understanding of the emotional and developmental needs of the child. Parent educators themselves require a broader understanding of child development and parent–child interactions, so that their support and input is less prescriptive and problem-focused and more facilitative of parents' own knowledge and understanding of their child. This in turn depends on the encouragement of a more genuine partnership between parents and professionals.

Support for parents and sharing understanding and ideas about child development, for parents as well as professionals, needs to be development-based rather than problem-based. Such an approach enables parents and professionals to develop a greater understanding of what behaviour is appropriate according to the age and circumstances of the child and what is not. A greater understanding of the *meaning* of children's behaviour will also help us to move away from a unidimensional approach to family problems and assist parents and professionals gain a greater understanding of how the problem originates. This would enable parents to move from a position of perpetual dependence on the expert to provide the answer to a degree of more appropriate independence of thought for themselves. It is an approach that is summed up by the classic phrase of an aid agency in the Third World that states that *you can give a hungry man a fish or you can teach him how to fish.*

Improved childcare arrangements

If parents are better informed about their child's developmental needs they will be better able to assess the quality of childcare for their children. Parents and professionals together need to be responsible for the kind of childcare arrangements they think would be best for infants and young children. It is not appropriate for parents to hand over all responsibility to childcare workers, kindergarten teachers and indeed to educationalists. They need to be helped to work in partnership. This requires that parents maintain a sense of responsibility themselves, as well as a sense of commitment and obligation to their children. For their part, it is vitally important that professionals do not de-skill parents and take over their responsibility. It is only in this way that parents and professionals can assess together what the young child needs. For example, in assessing optimum childcare arrangements the effects of an open-plan environment on young children can be realistically assessed by both parents and caregivers. Practical suggestions can then be made together about how the physical environment can be altered to better accommodate the children. Other important areas for sharing concerns include dealing with transitions and separations, asking what it might mean for the child when important carers come and go and explaining to parents that their child has had a difficult day. An open and honest approach to these realities works to mitigate blame, either of professionals or of parents and certainly of the child.

Advocating for changes to childcare

The work of childcare staff needs to be recognised as second in importance only to that of parents themselves. Raising the status, salaries and levels of training of those working in the childcare sector would acknowledge their important role. Staff in childcare centres are often at the forefront of identifying children at risk as well as children whose family and social relationships make them vulnerable to developing behavioural problems.

Urgent attention is needed to encourage the presence of positive male role models, particularly in the field of early childhood, to counter the experience for boys of growing up in an all-female world.

Supporting boys in tomorrow's society

The point has been made that boys are particularly vulnerable to being diagnosed as having ADHD and some of the psychological and social causations have been described. Again it is vital to view this as a problem that needs to have a link with the broader community rather than for clinicians, teachers and childcare workers to struggle to fill the gap because of broader societal indifference or lack of attention.

It is a problem that in fact requires to be better understood by men themselves and by fathers. Biddulph (1994) makes the point that women teachers in particular need to be 'released from the need to fight with problem boys'. He says that these boys are hungry for fathering and 'need to be engaged, valued and disciplined by strong loving male figures'. One could argue for a similar release for many mothers who struggle to bring up boys single-handedly, even though a father might be present in the home. Biddulph recommends introducing the concept of training male teachers in a mentor role. Such training would necessarily include education in human development, counselling and conflict resolution.

Addressing the current crisis for boys might require that we bring the problem home directly to men in the workplace where men and fathers spend much of their time. Traditionally the artificial split between home and work can provide justification for fathers' lack of involvement. However, the point needs to be made that the boys who have difficulty with attention and capacity to learn today will be the employees of tomorrow.

Government bodies, trades unions and companies thus have a responsibility towards the next generation. They must ensure that the vital task of fatherhood is not only supported and valued, but that fathers can be 'released' to their families—that is allowed an appropriate time frame in which to contribute to the basic mental health of their children.

Identifying risks—working preventively

Taking a broader view of the problem of ADD and ADHD enables professionals to better identify clusters of 'risk factors' at an early age and early stage.

McIntosh (1997), in a review of the research on the practices that promote wellbeing in child development, makes the point that 'a focus on early prevention of difficulties through strategies aimed at the individual parents, family and community are likely to promote positive patterns of emotional and behavioural health in children. The concept of promotion then seems inextricably linked with the tasks of prevention' (p. 9).

McIntosh explores the practical implications for promoting what are described as 'pro-social' behaviours in childhood. She refers to the research of Hawkins and Catalano (1996), which confirms the importance of a multidisciplinary and multiple-intervention approach to reducing the problem of antisocial behaviour. Hawkins and Catalano emphasise the need to gear the primary socialising units of the child at their specific developmental level through parent education, school intervention, community programs and social policy developments.

Of particular relevance to the subject of ADD and ADHD is McIntosh's conclusion to her review of the literature, which indicates that there are two key developmental tasks that must be achieved in early childhood to lower the risk of future mental health problems. These are:

- the acquisition of language skills to prepare the child to read and write;
- the development of impulse control.

Failure at these tasks has been associated with later behavioural and school maladjustment and with the development of mental health problems (Hawkins & Catalano, 1992, p. 27).

McIntosh emphasises the multi-factorial elements in child mental health problems. She states that in considering childhood antisocial behaviour and its prevention, one is inevitably drawn to consider the problems of attachment disturbance, learning difficulties and poor social skills. In exploring the prevention of childhood depression we must similarly take a preventive view of the impact of socioeconomic factors, family hardship, maternal depression, child abuse and neglect and learning and neurological difficulties. She confirms the view we have reiterated throughout this book that 'it is important to bear in mind the depth and dimensions behind any one disorder, let alone any one child's difficulties and the labyrinth of connections between the risk and resilience factors that define them' (McIntosh, 1997, p. 25).

Developing public health preventive interventions—some examples

In Australia the 'High Risk Infant' initiative run by the Department of Human Services is a good example of putting in place a strong preventive strategy for the most vulnerable families in the population.

There are a number of new initiatives being trialled (McIntosh, 1997) to promote the early detection and prevention of developmental and behavioural difficulties. In one such initiative the plan is to develop a methodology such as a questionnaire whereby parents can communicate their concerns about their children to 'front line professionals' such as maternal and child health nurses, childcare workers and pre-school teachers. In the United States, the Touchpoints Program (Stadtler et al., 1995) directly utilises a developmental approach by setting up parent groups at predictable times in the infant and young child's development that represent growth points or changes within the child and that have a resultant impact on their behaviour, and indeed on the family. The task of the facilitator of each group is not to provide an answer but to encourage the sharing and support of the group participants. Providing insight in the emotional experience of the developing child is one of the aims of the group.

The positive outcome of good early intervention is demonstrated by a number of longitudinal outcome studies in the United States, for example the Carolina Abecedarian Project, which was part of an experimental educational intervention between 1972 and 1985 (Shore, 1997). This project served children from low-income families from early infancy through to the primary school years. The services included high-quality full-day childcare and regular support and education for parents. The infant curriculum was designed to enhance cognitive language, perceptual motor and social development. In the later pre-school years there was an emphasis on pre-literacy skills and language development. The follow-up assessments conducted at ages eight, twelve and fifteen found that this program had a positive effect on children's intellectual development and academic achievement. These positive results continued through to ages twelve and fifteen, where it was found that the children who had participated in the service had IQ scores that were on average 5.3 points higher than a comparative group of non-participants. These higher achievement scores were maintained at age fifteen.

Other projects in the United States, such as the High/Scope Perry pre-school project (Shore, 1997) have focused on the provision of intensive pre-school programs for three- and four-year-olds, which included health and family support services. Since the start of the study in 1963, researchers have tracked a number of indicators as part of the ongoing longitudinal study. These include juvenile delinquency, utilisation of special education services, arrests, teenage pregnancy, post-secondary education and employment history. The follow-up study of participants at the age of 27 found that the children who had participated in the early childhood program did significantly better than a comparison group on all of these indicators.

Dealing with the aftermath of separation and divorce

As we have stated in Chapter 4, the experience of separation and divorce has a potentially disruptive and destabilising effect on children, particularly when they feel under pressure to make choices that are beyond their capacity and control. Encouraging greater access on the part of the non-custodial parent and their more positive involvement in the lives of their children is crucial, particularly for boys and their fathers. In Australia, the Federal Government's advisory body on family law has called for changes in the way parents negotiate arrangements regarding their children after divorce. The active encouragement of parents to set up a family plan that will be to the best benefit of the children appears to be a step in the right direction. However, parents at this vulnerable point in their lives require informed advice about the impact on children of different kinds of living arrangements. Again we have to keep in mind that the living arrangements that might suit working parents, involving 'rostering' the children between homes, might have a detrimental effect on those children's development.

Making positive changes to the school environment

Many children embark on the road to an ADD or ADHD diagnosis as a result of difficulties experienced within the school. These might be related to acting-out behaviour, to concentration or learning difficulties or all three. While we acknowledge the stresses teachers are under, little can be gained from demanding that parents seek an ADHD diagnosis for their child on the basis of this behaviour alone, when teachers are not informed about the family background or the stresses that the child might be experiencing.

On a day-to-day level there are a number of changes that can be made in the classroom that can have positive effects. For example, the traditional arrangements regarding the physical structure of the classroom and the use of 'chalk and talk' teaching present a hurdle for children with attention problems. Teachers need to become more aware of the classroom as a 'group' and of group dynamics within the classroom, which is quite different from viewing the class purely as a number of individuals. Understanding the dynamics of the group can throw light on, for example, how and why certain disruptive children always seem to get into trouble when in fact they might be used by those better behaved to cause diversions in the classroom.

Schmuck and Schmuck (1983) emphasise the importance of understanding the group processes in the classroom, which will stand children in good stead in later life since the increasing complexity of social life demands that we learn to work more effectively in groups. They believe that schools have a responsibility to help students develop behavioural and interpersonal skills concurrent with the academic curriculum. They introduce the concept of *classroom climate* to assist teachers to identify what is actually going on within the dynamics of the classroom. They state that classroom climate can be assessed by observing physical movement, bodily gestures, the handling of aggression and patterns of verbal interaction. The ease or reticence with which pupils interact with the teacher is also an indicator, as well as the way seating is organised. For example, do the seating arrangements shift from time to time to reflect different learning experiences or do they remain the same regardless of the learning activity?

The need to change and challenge conventional attitudes to teaching and learning requires that teachers for their part are also prepared to engage in a learning process and in some cases 'unlearn' what has been accepted conventional wisdom but might have outlived its usefulness. This is a process that cannot take place without appropriate training and support.

Bridging the gap between home and school

For many children under stress the split between home and school life is too difficult for them to bridge. The Healthy Families project referred to by McIntosh (1997), in which one of the authors (Schmidt Neven) was involved, attempted to bridge this gap with positive results. The state-based Healthy Families Project was managed by the Board of Studies and sponsored by the Health Promotion Foundation. It provided a Grade 6 classroom-based curriculum around family and emotional health that taught children to understand their own and other's families, and the ways that parenting patterns are transmitted across generations. The risk factors addressed in the project included stress and abuse within families, experiences of loss and separation and family discord.

The training program on child development designed by Schmidt Neven (1996) for the teaching staff as part of the pilot project included suggestions on how the classroom could be arranged more informally for this teaching module to enhance the communication between the teachers and the pupils. The training also focused on understanding group dynamics in the classroom in relation to the new curriculum, and on children sharing more personal information with their teachers and peers.

Evaluation of the pilot program revealed a high rate of satisfaction among teachers, pupils and parents. A particularly interesting finding was that following the teaching of this module, which encouraged the children to be more open about their lives at home, there appeared to be an improved degree of cohesion in the class group and communication improved overall, which had a positive effect on learning in other subjects (McIntosh, 1997). The outcome of this study suggests that younger children particularly have a need for a sense of connectedness between school and home and that this facilitates a sense of greater personal integration.

Conclusions

The recommendations made in this chapter reflect our view that ADHD is, in the majority of cases, a symptom of a breakdown in functioning for the child on a number of different levels, and that understanding, support and treatment need to reflect the complexity of this situation. In our recommendations we argue for a broad-based multidisciplinary approach from the professionals involved. We are also convinced that the identification of children with ADD and ADHD can most usefully lead us to review the potential for mental health for *all* children. We therefore include recommendations for changes within the settings and institutions that are responsible for the welfare of the child from the family through to education, the world of work, economics and government legislation as a step towards such health promotion. The promotion of a dialogue between these diverse groups as well as between professionals from different disciplines might lead to a level of collaboration that can do justice to the complexities of child and family mental health in the twenty-first century.

APPENDIX 1

DSM-IV Criteria for Attention Deficit Hyperactivity Disorder
(Reprinted with permission from Diagnostic and Statistical Manual of Mental disorders, Fourth Edition Text Revision. Copyright 2000 American Psychiatric Association.)

A. Either (1) or (2):

(1) Inattention: at least six of the following symptoms of inattention have persisted for at least six months to a degree that is maladaptive and inconsistent with developmental level:
(a) often fails to give close attention to details or makes careless mistakes in school work, work, or other activities;
(b) often has difficulty sustaining attention in tasks or play activities;
(c) often does not seem to listen to what is being said to him/her;
(d) often does not follow through on instructions and fails to finish school work, chores, or duties in the workplace (not due to oppositional behaviour or failure to understand instructions);
(e) often has difficulties organising tasks and activities;
(f) often avoids or strongly dislikes tasks (such as school work or homework) that require sustained mental effort;
(g) often loses things necessary for tasks or activities (e.g. school assignments, pencils, books, tools, or toys);
(h) is often easily distracted by extraneous stimuli;
(i) often forgetful in daily activities.

(2) Hyperactivity–Impulsivity: at least six of the following symptoms of hyperactivity–impulsivity have persisted for at least six months to a degree that is maladaptive and inconsistent with developmental level:

Hyperactivity:
(a) often fidgets with hands or feet or squirms in seat;
(b) often leaves seat in classroom or in other situations in which remaining seated is expected;
(c) often runs about or climbs excessively in situations where it is inappropriate (in adolescents or adults may be limited to subjective feelings of restlessness);
(d) often has difficulty playing or engaging in leisure activities quietly;
(e) often 'on the go' or often acts as if 'driven by a motor';
(f) often talks excessively.
Impulsivity:
(g) often blurts out answers to questions before the questions have been completed;
(h) often has difficulty awaiting turn;
(i) often interrupts or intrudes on other (e.g. butts into conversations or games).

B. Some hyperactive–impulsive or inattentive symptoms that caused impairment were present before age seven years.

C. Some impairment from symptoms is present in two or more settings (e.g. at school, work, and at home).

D. There must be clear evidence of clinically significant impairment in social, academic, or occupational functioning.

E. The symptoms do not occur exclusively during the course of Personality Disorder, Schizophrenia, or other Psychotic Disorder, and are not better accounted for by another mental disorder (e.g. Mood Disorder, Anxiety Disorder, Dissociative Disorder, or a Personality Disorder).

APPENDIX 2

ICD-10 Classification of Mental and Behavioural Disorders Criteria (World Health Organization, 1993)

F90 Hyperkinetic disorders

G1 Inattention
At least six of the following symptoms of attention have persisted for at least six months, to a degree that is maladaptive and inconsistent with the developmental level of the child:
(1) often fails to give close attention to details, or makes careless errors in school work, work or other activities;
(2) often fails to sustain attention in tasks or play activities;
(3) often appears not to listen to what is being said to him or her;
(4) often fails to follow through on instructions or to finish school work, chores, or duties in the workplace (not because of oppositional behaviour or failure to understand instructions);
(5) is often impaired in organising tasks and activities;
(6) often avoids or strongly dislikes tasks, such as homework, that require sustained mental effort;
(7) often loses things necessary for certain tasks and activities, such as school assignments, pencils, books, toys or tools;
(8) is often easily distracted by external stimuli;
(9) is often forgetful in the course of daily activities.

G2 Hyperactivity
At least three of the following symptoms of hyperactivity have persisted for at least six months, to a degree that is maladaptive and inconsistent with the developmental level of the child:

(1) often fidgets with hands or feet or squirms on seat;
(2) leaves seat in classroom or in other situations in which remaining seated is expected;
(3) often runs about or climbs excessively in situations in which it is inappropriate (in adolescents or adults, only feelings of restlessness may be present);
(4) is often unduly noisy in playing or has difficulty in engaging quietly in leisure activities;
(5) exhibits a persistent pattern of excessive motor activity that is not substantially modified by social context or demands.

G3 Impulsivity

At least one of the following symptoms of impulsivity has persisted for at least six months, to a degree that is maladaptive and inconsistent with the developmental level of the child:

(1) often blurts out answers before questions have been completed;
(2) often fails to wait in lines or await turns in games or group situations;
(3) often interrupts or intrudes on others (e.g. butts into others' conversations or games);
(4) often talks excessively without appropriate response to social constraints.

G4

Onset of the disorder is no later than the age of seven years.

G5 Pervasiveness

The criteria should be met for more than a single situation, e.g. the combination of inattention and hyperactivity should be present both at home and at school, or at both school and another setting where children are observed, such as a clinic. (Evidence for cross-situationality will ordinarily require information from more than one source; parental reports about classroom behaviour, for instance, are unlikely to be sufficient.)

G6

The symptoms in G1–G3 cause clinically significant distress or impairment in social, academic, or occupational functioning.

G7
The disorder does not meet the criteria for pervasive developmental disorders (F84.–), manic episode (F30.–), depressive episode (F32.–), or anxiety disorders (F41.–).

Comment
Many authorities also recognise conditions that are sub-threshold for hyperkinetic disorder. Children who meet criteria in other ways but do not show abnormalities of hyperactivity/impulsiveness may be recognised as showing attention deficit; conversely, children who fall short of criteria for attention problems but meet criteria in other respects may be recognised as showing activity disorder. In the same way, children who meet criteria for only one situation (e.g. only the home or only the classroom) may be regarded as showing a home-specific or classroom-specific disorder. These conditions are not yet included in the main classification because of insufficient empirical predictive validation, and because many children with sub-threshold disorders show other syndromes (such as Oppositional Defiant Disorder, F91.3) and should be classified in the appropriate category.

F90.0 Disturbance of activity and attention
The general criteria for hyperkinetic disorder (F90) must be met, but not those for conduct disorders (F91.–).

F90.1 Hyperkinetic Conduct Disorder
The general criteria for both hyperkinetic disorder (F90) and conduct disorders (F91.–) must be met.

F90.8 Other hyperkinetic disorder

F90.9 Hyperkinetic disorder, unspecified
This residual category is not recommended and should be used only when there is a lack of differentiation between F90.0 and F90.1, but the overall criteria for F90.– are fulfilled.

Glossary

Many of the terms explained below will be familiar to health professionals. This glossary is intended as an aid to interested non-professionals and professionals working outside the health sciences.

aetiology   the cause of a medical condition

autonomic nervous system   that part of the nervous system that is responsible for effecting action on the internal environment of the body; it does so via muscles (e.g. heart muscle) and glands (e.g. salivary glands)

axon   part of a neuron consisting of a long extension that transmits outgoing electrochemical impulses to other neurons

basal ganglia   a group of subcortical brain nuclei that function in the integration and coordination of information from higher or lower brain regions; includes caudate/putamen (also called striatum) and globus pallidus

biological marker   a measurable physical symptom that can be isolated as the cause of a condition

biomedical perspective   the view that health and illness results from the action of discrete biological factors

biopsychosocial perspective   the view that health and illness result from the complex interaction between biological, psychological and social factors in people's lives

cognitive functioning   the ability to perform cognitive processing tasks

comorbidity   the presence of two or more disorders in an individual at the same time

continuous performance tests computerised tasks that are continuously presented over an extended time frame so as to assess a child's ability to sustain attention and refrain from impulsive responding

dendrite a branched protoplasmic process of a neuron that conducts impulses to the cell body. There are usually several to a cell. They form synaptic connections with other neurons

dopamine a chemical or 'neurotransmitter' in the brain. It is called a neurotransmitter because it carries or transmits messages between nerves in the brain. Dopamine is sent from one nerve and is then received on another nerve by a 'receptor'. The receptors for dopamine are called 'dopamine receptors'

dopamine transporter the protein on the surface of dopamine neurons that takes up dopamine after it has been released into the synapse in order to terminate its effect

dopamine type 4 receptor one of five subtypes of the receptor for dopamine

DSM criteria the qualitative criteria that need to be met for a person to qualify for a psychiatric label from the Diagnostic and Statistical Manual of the American Psychiatric Association

EEG (electroencephalography) a record obtained by attaching electrodes to the scalp and amplifying the spontaneous electrical activity of the brain. Familiar aspects of the EEG are alpha waves (8–13 Hz) and delta waves of slower frequency

eugenics the movement, popular in the early part of the twentieth century, that sought to increase the quality of human genetic stock by selective breeding

evoked potentials an electrical discharge in some part of the nervous system produced by stimulation elsewhere. The measured potential is commonly based on response averaging by a computer

executive functions the cognitive abilities necessary for complex goal-directed behaviour and adaptation to a range of environmental changes and demands. Functions include ability to plan and anticipate outcomes (cognitive flexibility), to direct attentional resources to meet the demands of non-routine events, self-monitoring and self-awareness necessary for *appropriateness* of behaviour and behavioural flexibility

factor analysis a complex statistical technique based on correlation and used to calculate the number and nature of factors within a test

foetal alcohol syndrome (FAS) occurs after substantial alcohol exposure in utero and is characterised by facial dysmorphic features, poor growth, microcephaly, mental retardation and disturbed attention

fragile x syndrome an x-linked syndrome caused by a fragile site on the x chromosome. Clinical features in males include mental retardation, hyperactivity, characteristic facial dysmorphic features and large testicles (after puberty)

frontal lobe one of the four lobes of the brain. It includes all the cortex that lies anterior to the central sulcus and superior to the lateral fissure. It is divided into motor, premotor and prefrontal areas. The prefrontal cortex is anterior to the prefrontal area and is the largest of the three divisions. This latter area is concerned with executive functions, and many other cognitive functions

globus pallidus one of the three nuclei that make up the basal ganglia. It relays information from the caudate and putamen (the neostriatum) to the thalamus and the frontal cortex. It is sometimes called the pallidum

halo effect an appraisal error owing to generalisation from one positive or negative characteristic to other ones

heterogeneous condition a condition that has no single cause and comprises a number of distinct elements

homogeneous all of the same kind

hyperkinetic overactive and characterised by excessive movement

learning disability a group of disorders manifested by significant difficulties in the acquisition and use of listening, speaking, reading, writing, reasoning or mathematical abilities

medical model the view that illness results exclusively from biological factors and bodily processes

MRI (magnetic resonance imaging) a procedure in which the brain is exposed to a strong magnetic field that momentarily affects the spin of the hydrogen atoms in the water molecules within the brain cells. When the atoms return to their normal spin they release detectable signals that can be captured as computer-generated images. The result is a detailed picture of the brain's soft tissue

neurology the medical specialty that focuses on conditions affecting the nervous system

neuron the nerve cell; the basic unit of the synaptic nervous system

neuropsychology an applied science devoted to the examination of relationships between brain dysfunction and behaviour *neurotransmitter*   a chemical involved in the transmission of nerve impulses across the synapse from one neuron to another. Usually released from small vesicles in the synaptic terminals of the axon in response to the action potential; diffuses across the synapse to influence electrical activity in another neuron

norm-referenced measures   assessment instruments indicating how an individual is functioning in relation to peers with similar background characteristics

oppositional defiant disorder   one of the disruptive behaviour disorders characterised by at least four symptoms such as having a bad temper; blaming others; arguing; annoying others and being easily annoyed; actively defying; and frequently being angry, spiteful or vindictive

paediatric neuropsychologists   specialists in the provision of clinical and research services to children and adolescents, mostly concerning medical syndromes that alter the normal functioning of the nervous system. Practitioners in this field tend to have a strong background in developmental psychology and cognitive psychology, as well as extensive neurological knowledge of brain growth and function. As a professional group, they are often consulted by other psychologists, psychiatrists, doctors, neurologists and neurosurgeons to assist in the identification of underlying neurological disorders

pathology   the science of bodily disease

pathology-based perspective   a way of looking at a person that focuses on what is diseased

pervasive developmental disorder   a group of disorders characterised by impairments in language, communicative and social functioning, associated with a restricted repertoire of activities; includes autism, childhood disintegrative disorder, Asperger's syndrome, Rett's syndrome

PET (positron emission tomography)   a computer-based scanning procedure that measures the radioactivity of glucose molecules to map metabolic activities of the living brain during cognitive tasks

prefrontal cortex   the cortical region in the frontal lobe that is anterior to the primary and association motor cortices. It is thought to be involved in planning complex cognitive behaviours and in the expression of personality and appropriate social behaviour. It is divided into the dorsolateral, orbitofrontal (also called the limbic frontal lobe) and mesial prefrontal areas

psychodynamic approach an approach which emphasises the emotional content and meaning of all human experience and the importance of relationships in the formation of personality. In this book a psychodynamic approach is presented which promotes links between individual development, the family, the organization and the community. While a psychodynamic approach is traditionally associated with psychotherapy, it has applications well beyond the treatment modality. A psychodynamic approach can be utilised in a wide range of settings such as education, health care, early child development and the work force to promote greater understanding of behaviour in everyday life.

psychometric tests carefully constructed and standardised measures of psychological characteristics possessing reliability and validity

psychophysiological measures indicators of psychological processes or states, by measuring physiological determinants. In the end, the outcome of the physiological measures needs to be interpreted psychologically, and often related to psychological measures

psychosocial interventions ways of approaching childhood disturbances that focus on changing the psychological or social environment of the child. They can be contrasted with biological approaches, which aim to alter the chemical environment within the child

psychostimulant a drug that acts on the central nervous system to increase responsiveness

public health a focus on the factors in society, the environment and human behaviour that contribute to health and help prevent illness. Public health aims at creating healthy people and healthy communities, and works at improving the factors that make people sick. It encompasses health promotion, health education, environmental health, community development, health policy and research

self-regulation a term with a variety of interpretations within psychology but when used in a neuropsychological context it usually refers to the ability to choose a response and act successfully towards a goal. Children with ADHD experience difficulties inhibiting inappropriate behaviour and being able to consider alternative responses. They have difficulty changing their response when confronted with new data and are dogged by impulsivity.

The concept of self regulation provides a promising framework for an understanding of ADHD as it emphasises the essential psychosomatic nature of all human functioning. Thus it goes beyond the more linear focus of a purely medical approach. For example in the book we refer to the research evidence which explores the impact of disturbed and traumatic emotional experience on the development of the brain and immune system particularly in infancy and early childhood

structured interviews   a highly systematic format for conducting clinical interviews that facilitates diagnostic decision making using classification systems such as the DSM-IV

synapse   the point of junction between two neurons in a neural pathway, where the termination of the axon of one neuron comes into close proximity with the cell body or dendrites of another. At this point, where the relationship of the two neurons is one of contact only, the impulse travelling in the first neuron initiates an impulse in the second neuron. Synapses are polarised, i.e. the impulses pass in one direction only. They are susceptible to fatigue, offer a resistance to the passage of impulses and are markedly susceptible to the effects of oxygen deficiency, anaesthetics and other agents, including therapeutic drugs and toxic chemicals

Tourette's syndrome   the most complex tic disorder, characterised by multiple motor tics and at least one vocal tic

unidimensional condition   a psychiatric illness that comprises of only one aspect so that a person can be described completely in terms of how much of that single pathology they possess

vigilance   the ability to maintain alertness continuously without 'tuning out'. It is also called sustained attention

References

ABC Radio (2000). *The Health Report*, 23 October

Abikoff, H., Courtney, M., Pelham, W. & Koplewicz, H. (1994). Detection bias in teachers' ratings of attention deficit hyperactivity disorder and oppositional defiant disorder. *Journal of Abnormal Child Psychology*, 21 (5), pp. 519–33

Achenbach, T.M. (1991). *Manual for the Child Behavior Checklist*. University of Vermont, Burlington, Vermont, pp. 4–18

Achenbach, T. M. & Edelbrock, C. S. (1981). Behavioral problems and competencies reported by parents of normal and disturbed children aged four through sixteen. *Monographs of the Society for Research in Child Development*, 46, pp. 1–82

Achenbach, T. M., McConaughy, J. H. & Howell, C. T. (1987). Child/adolescent behavioural and emotional problems: Implications of cross-informant correlations for situational specificity. *Psychological Bulletin*, 101, pp. 213–32

Ahadpour, M., Horton, A. M. & Vaeth, J. M. (1993). Attention deficit disorder and drug abuse. *International Journal of Neuroscience*, 72 (1–2), pp. 89–93

Ainsworth, M., Blehar, M., Waters, E. & Walls, S. (1978). *Patterns of Attachment: A psychological study of the Strange Situation*. Lawrence Erlbaum Associates, Hillsdale, New Jersey

American Psychiatric Association (2000). *Diagnostic and Statistical Manual of Mental Disorders*, 4th Edition, Text Revision. American Psychiatric Association, Washington, D.C.

——(1994). *Diagnostic and Statistical Manual of Mental Disorders* (4th edn). American Psychiatric Association, Washington, D.C.

Anderson, J. C., Williams, S., McGee, R. & Silva, P. A. (1987). DSM-III disorders in preadolescent children: Prevalence in a large sample from the general population. *Archives of General Psychiatry*, 44, pp. 69–76

Anderson, V. (1998). Assessing executive functions in children: Biological, psychological, and developmental considerations. *Neuropsychological Rehabilitation*, 8 (3), pp. 319–49

Anderson, V. & Pentland, L. (1998). Residual attention deficits following childhood head injury: Implications for ongoing development. *Neuropsychological Rehabilitation*, 8 (3), pp. 283–300

Armstrong, L. (1993). *And They Call It Help: The psychiatric policing of America's children*. Addison-Wesley Publishing Company, Reading, Massachusetts

Armstrong, T. (1995). *The Myth of the A.D.D Child*. Dutton, New York

Bain, A. & Barnett, L. (1980). *The Design of a Day Care System in a Nursery Setting for Children under Five*. Final Report, Tavistock Institute of Human Relations, Doc. No. 2347

Bain, L. (1991). *A Parent's Guide to Attention Deficit Disorders*. Dell Publishing, New York

Baker, G. B., Bornstein, R. A., Douglass, A. B., Van Muyden, J. C., Ashton, S. & Bazylewich, T. L. (1993). Urinary excretion of MHPG and Normetanephrine in Attention Deficit Hyperactivity Disorder. *Molecular and Chemical Neuropathology*, 18 (1–2), pp. 173–8

Barkley, R. A. (1987). The assessment of Attention Deficit-Hyperactivity Disorder. *Behavioural Assessment*, 9, pp. 207–33

—— (1990). *Attention Deficit Disorder: A handbook for diagnosis and treatment*. Guilford Press, New York

—— (1992). The ecological validity of laboratory and analogue assessment methods of ADHD symptoms. *Journal of Abnormal Child Psychology*, 19, pp. 149–78

—— (1996). Critical issues in research on attention. In G. R. Lyon & N. A. Krasnegor (eds). *Attention, Memory and Executive Function*. Paul H. Brookes Publishing Co., Baltimore, pp. 45–56

—— (1997a). *ADHD and the Nature of Self-control*. Guilford, New York

—— (1997b). Attention deficit/hyperactivity disorder, self-regulation and time: Toward a more comprehensive theory. *Journal of Development and Behavioral Pediatrics*, 18 (4), pp. 271–9

—— (1997c). Behavioral inhibition, sustained attention, and executive functions: Constructing a unifying theory of ADHD. *Psychological Bulletin*, 121 (1), pp. 65–94

—— (1998a). *Attention Deficit Disorder: A handbook for diagnosis and treatment.* (2nd edn). Guilford Press, New York

—— (1998b). Attention-deficit-hyperactivity disorder. *Scientific American,* September

Baum, F. (1998). *The New Public Health: An Australian perspective.* Oxford University Press, South Melbourne

Baumeister, R. F., Heatherton, T. F. & Tice, D. M. (1994). *Losing Control: How and why people fail at self-regulation.* Academic Press, San Diego

Bertalanffy, L. von. (1973). *General System Theory.* Penguin, Harmondsworth

Biddulph, S. (1994). *Manhood.* Finch Publishing, Sydney

Biederman, J., Milberger, S., Faraone, S. V., Kiely, K., Guite, J., Mick, E., Ablon, S., Warburton, R. & Reed, E. (1995). Family environment risk factors for attention-deficit hyperactivity disorder. *Archives of General Psychiatry.* 52, pp. 464–70

Biederman, J., Newcorn, J. & Sprich, S. (1991). Comorbidity of attention deficit hyperactivity disorder with conduct, depressive, anxiety, and other disorders. *American Journal of Psychiatry,* 148, pp. 564–77

Billington, T. (1996). Pathologising children: Psychology in education and acts of government. In Erica Burman et al. *Psychology discourse practice: From regulation to resistance.* Taylor & Francis Ltd, London U.K. pp. 37–54

Bion, W. R. (1964). Container and contained. In *Attention and Interpretation.* W. Heinemann, London, pp. 72–82; Karnac Books, London (1993)

Blankenhorn, D. (1995). *Fatherless America: Confronting our most urgent social problem.* Harper Perennial, New York

Boston, M. & Szur, R. (eds). (1983). *Psychotherapy with Severely Deprived Children.* Routledge & Kegan Paul, London; reprinted Karnac Books, London (1990)

Bowlby, J. (1973a). *Attachment.* Penguin, Harmondsworth

—— (1973b). *Separation.* Penguin, Harmondsworth

—— (1973c). *Loss.* Penguin, Harmondsworth

—— (1988). *A Secure Base: Clinical applications of attachment theory.* Routledge, London

Bradley, C. (1937). The behaviour of children receiving Benzedrine. *American Journal of Psychiatry,* 94, pp. 577–85. Referred to in The British Psychological Society (1996). *Attention Deficit Hyper-*

activity Disorder (ADHD): A psychological response to an evolving concept, p. 14

Brazelton, T. B. (1992). *Touchpoints*. Penguin, London

Brazelton, T. B. & Cramer, B. G. (1990). *The Earliest Relationship: Parents, infants and the drama of early attachment*. Addison-Wesley, Reading, Mass

Breggin, P. R. (1994). *The War against Children: How drugs, programs and theories of the psychiatric establishment are threatening America's children with a medical 'cure' for violence*. St. Martin's Press, New York

—— (1997). *Brain Disabling Treatments in Psychiatry: Drugs, electroshock and the role of the FDA*. Springer, New York

—— (1998). *Talking Back to Ritalin*. Common Courage Press, New York

—— (1999). Psychostimulants in the treatment of children diagnosed with ADHD: Part 1—Acute risks and psychological effects. *Ethical Human Sciences and Services*, 1 (1), pp. 13–33

British Psychological Society. (1996). *Attention Deficit Hyperactivity Disorder (ADHD): A psychological response to an evolving concept*. The British Psychological Society, London

Bronfenbrenner, U. (1986). Ecology of the family as a context for human development: Research perspectives. *Developmental Psychology*, 22, pp. 723–42

Brown, R. T., Madan-Swain, A. & Baldwin, K. (1991). Gender differences in a clinic-referred sample of attention-deficit disordered children. *Child Psychiatry and Human Development*, 22, pp. 111–29

Campbell, S. B., Pierce, E. W., March, C. L., Ewing, L .J. & Szumowski, E. E. (1994). Hard to manage preschoolers: Symptomatic behavior across contexts and time. *Child Development*, 65, pp. 836–51

Cantwell, D. P. & Hanna, G. L. (1989). Attention Deficit Hyperactivity Disorder. In A. Tasman, R. E. Hales & A. J. Francis (eds). *Review of Psychiatry*, pp. 134–61

Castellanos, F.X. (1996). Quantitative Brain Magnetic Resonance Imaging in Attention Deficit Hyperactivity Disorder. *Archives of General Psychiatry*, 53, pp. 605–16

Castellanos, F. X., Giedd, J. N., Eckburg, P., Marsh, W. L., Vaituzis, A. C., Kaysen, A. C., Hamburger, S. D. & Rapoport, J. L. (1994). Quantitative morphology of the caudate nucleus in attention deficit hyperactivity disorder. *American Journal of Psychiatry*, 151 (12), pp. 1791–6

Catalano, R. & Hawkins, J. D. (1996). The social development model: A theory of antisocial behaviour. In J. David Hawkins (ed.). *Delinquency and Crime: Current theories*. Cambridge University Press, Cambridge. Referred to in J. McIntosh (1997). *Promoting Well Being in Child Development: A review of recent literature research and practices*. Victorian Health Promotion Foundation Series, Australia, p. 17

Catroppa, C., Anderson V. & Stargatt, R. (1999). A prospective analysis of the recovery of attention following pediatric head injury. *Journal of the International Neuropsychological Society*, 5, pp. 48–57

Chess, S. & Thomas, A. (1989). Issues in the clinical application of temperament. In G. A. Kohnstamm, J. E. Bates & M. K. Rothbart (eds). *Temperament in Childhood*. John Wiley & Sons, New York

Clulow, C. F. (1982). *To Have and To Hold: Marriage, the first baby and preparing couples for parenthood*. Aberdeen University Press, Aberdeen

Cockett, M. & Tripp, J. (1994). *The Exeter Family Study: Family breakdown and its impact on children*. University of Exeter Press, Exeter

Conner, D. F. (1998). Other medications in the treatment of child and adolescent ADHD. In R. A. Barkley (ed.). *Attention Deficit Disorder: A handbook for diagnosis and treatment* (2nd edn). Guilford Press, New York

Conners, C. K. (1995). *Conners Continuous Performance Test User's Manual*. Multi-Health Systems, Toronto, Canada

— (1997). *The Conners Rating Scales: Instruments for the assessment of childhood psychopathology*. Children's Hospital National Medical Center, Washington, DC

Cooley, E. L. & Morris, R. D. (1990). Attention in children: A neuropsychologically based model for assessment. *Developmental Neuropsychology*, 6, pp. 239–74

Cooper, P. (1998). Developments in the Understanding of Childhood Emotional and Behavioural Problems Since 1981. In R. Laslett, P. Cooper, P. Maras, A. Rimmer & B. Law (eds). *Changing Perceptions: Emotional and behavioural difficulties since 1945*. The Association of Workers for Children with Emotional and Behavioural Difficulties, Kent

Cunningham, C. E. (1999). In the wake of the MTA: Charting a new course for the study and treatment of attention deficit disorder. *Canadian Journal of Psychiatry*, 44, pp. 999–1006

Davies, S. (1996). Letter to the editors. *Journal of Child Psychotherapy*, 22 (2), under Correspondence, pp. 315–17

Davis, M. & Walbridge, D. (1981). *Boundary and Space: An introduction to the work of D. W. Winnicott*. Karnac Books, London

Daws, D. (1989). *Through the Night: Helping parents and sleepless infants*. Free Association Books, London

Delaney, J., Lupton, M. & Toth, E. (1988). *The Curse*. University of Illinois Press, Urbana and Chicago

Denckla, M. B. (1989). Executive function, the overlap zone between attention deficit disorder and learning disabilities. *International Paediatrics*, 4 (2), pp. 155–60

—— (1991). Attention Deficit Hyperactivity Disorder—Residual type. *Journal of Child Neurology*, 6, S44–50

Dickman, S. J. (1993). Impulsivity and information processing. In W. G. McCown, J. L. Johnson & M. B. Shure (eds). *The Impulsive Client: Theory, research, and treatment*. American Psychological Society, Washington, pp. 151–84

Diller, L. H. (1990). Running on Ritalin. *Double Take*, Bantam, U.S.

Douglas, V. I. (1972). Stop, look, listen: The problem of sustained attention and impulse control in hyperactive and normal children. *Canadian Journal of Behavioural Science*, 4, pp. 259–82

—— (1983). Attention and cognitive problems. In M. Rutter (ed.). *Developmental Neuropsychiatry*. Guilford Press, New York

Douglas, V. I. & Peters, K. G. (1979). Toward a clear definition of the attentional deficit of hyperactive children. In G. A. Hale & M. Lewis (eds). *Attention and the Development of Cognitive Skills*. Plenum, New York, pp. 173–248

Draeger, S., Prior, M. & Sanson, A. (1986). Visual and auditory attention performance in hyperactive children: Competence or compliance. *Journal of Abnormal Child Psychology*, 14, pp. 411–24

Early Childhood Research Network (2000). Child Care and Children's Peer Interaction at 24 and 36 months. *Child Development*, 72, pp. 1478–1500

Eaves, L., Silberg, J., Hewitt, J. K., Meyer, J., Rutter, M., Sononoff, S., Neale, M. & Pickles, A. (1993). Genes, personality and psychopathology: A latent class analysis of hereditary liability symptoms of attention deficit hyperactivity disorder in twins. In R. Plomin & G. E. McClearn (eds). *Nature, Nurture and Psychology*. APA Books, Washington, DC

Emde, R. N. (1987). Development terminable and interminable.

Paper presented at the 35th International Psychoanalytical Congress. July, Montreal, Canada

Engel, G. L. (1977). The need for a new medical model: A challenge for biomedicine. *Science*, 196, pp. 129–36

—— (1980). The clinical application of the biopsychosocial model. *American Journal of Psychiatry*, 137, pp. 355–544

Engelmann, S. & Carnine, D. (1982). *Theory of Instruction: Principles and applications*. Irvington, New York

Erickson, M., Sroufe, L. A. & Egeland, B. (1985). The relationship between quality of attachment and behavior problems in pre-school in a high risk sample. In I. Bretherton & E. Waters (eds). Growing points of attachment theory and research. *Monographs for the Society for Research in Child Development*. 50 (Nos. 1–2), pp. 147–66

Erskine, A. & Judd, D. (1994). *The Imaginative Body: Psychodynamic therapy in health care*. Whurr Publications, London

Eyestone, L. L. & Howell, R. J. (1994). An epidemiological study of attention deficit hyperactivity disorder and major depression in a male prison population. *Bulletin of the American Academy of Psychiatry and the Law*, 22 (2), pp. 181–93

Fajerman, L., Jarrett, M. & Sutton, F. (2000). *Children As Partners in Planning: A training resource to support consultation with children*. Save the Children, UK

Faraone, S. V. (1996). Discussion of: Genetic influence on parent reported attention-related problems in a Norwegian general population twin sample. *Journal of the American Academy of Child and Adolescent Psychiatry*, 35, pp. 586–98

Fergusson, D. M., Lynskey, M. T. & Horwood, L. J. (1993). The effect of maternal depression on maternal ratings of child behaviour. *Journal of Abnormal Child Psychology*. 21, pp. 245–70

Forehand, R., Wierson, M., Frame, C., Kempton, T. & Armistead, L. (1991). Juvenile delinquency entry and persistence: Do attention problems contribute to conduct problems? *Journal of Behavior Therapy and Experimental Psychiatry*, 22 (4), pp.. 261–4

Foucault, M. (1965). *Madness and Civilization: A history of insanity in the age of reason*. (R. Howard trans.). Tavistock, London

Fraiberg, S. (1959). *The Magic Years: Understanding and handling the problems of early childhood*. Charles Scribner & Sons/Macmillan,

—— (ed.) (1980). *Clinical Studies in Infant Mental Health: The first year of life*. Tavistock, London

Furman, R. (1996). Letter to the editors. *Journal of Child Psychotherapy*, 22 (1), under Correspondence, pp. 157–160

Garton, A., Farrelly, J., Anderson, V., Pawsey, R. & Standish, J. (1997). *Attention Deficit Hyperactivity Disorder in Children: A guide to best practice for psychologists*. Australian Psychological Society.

Goodman, R. & Stevenson, J. (1989). A twin study of hyperactivity—II: The aetiological role of genes, family relationships and peri-natal adversity. *Journal of Child Psychology and Psychiatry*, 30, pp. 691–709

Grainger, J. (1997). *Children's Behaviour, Attention and Reading Problems*. ACER, Melbourne

Gray, J. (1999). The myth of progress. Saturday essay, *The Age*, Melbourne, 8 May

Green, M., Wong, M., Atkins, D., et al. (1999). *Diagnosis of Attention Deficit/Hyperactivity Disorder: Technical Review 3*. US Department of Health and Human Services, Agency for Health Care Policy and Research, Rockville, MD

Greenberg, L. M. and Waldman, I. D. (1993). Developmental normative data on the test of variables of attention (TOVA). *Journal of Child Psychology and Psychiatry*, 34, pp. 1019–34

Gunnar, M. R. (1996). Quality of care and the buffering of stress physiology: Its potential in protecting the developing human brain. University of Minnesota Institute of Child Development. Cited in Shore (1997), pp. 28–9

Hagerman, R. J., Jackson, C., Amiri, K., Silverman, A. C., O'Connor, R. & Sobesky, W. (1992). Girls with fragile X syndrome: Physical and neurocognitive status and outcome. *Pediatrics*, 89 (3), pp. 395–400

Halperin, J. M. (1996). Conceptualizing, describing, and measuring components of attention: A summary. In G. R. Lyon & N. A. Krasnegor (eds). *Attention, Memory, and Executive Function*, Paul Brooks Publishing Co., Baltimore, pp. 119–36

Halperin, J. M., Matier, K., Bedi, G., Sharma, V. & Newcorn, J. H. (1992). Specificity of inattention, impulsivity and hyperactivity to the diagnosis of attention deficit hyperactivity disorder. *Journal of the American Academy of Child and Adolescent Psychiatry*, 31 (2), pp. 190–6

Hawkins, D., Catalano, R., Morrison, D., O'Donnell, J. Abbott, R. and Day, L. E. (1992). The Seattle Social Development Project: Effects of the first four years on protective factors and problem behaviours. In J. McCord and R. Tremblay (eds). *Preventing Antisocial Behaviour: Interventions from birth through adolescence*. Guilford Press, New York. Referred to in J. McIntosh (1997).

Promoting Well Being in Child Development: A review of recent literature research and practices. Victorian Health Promotion Foundation Series, Australia, p. 27

Hazell, P. (2000). Attention Deficit Hyperactivity Disorder in preschool aged children. Vol. 1 in R. Kosky, A. O'Hanlon, G. Martin & C. Davis (series eds). *Clinical Approaches to Early Intervention in Child and Adolescent Mental Health.* Australian Early Intervention Network for Mental Health in Young People, (AusEinet), Commonwealth of Australia, Adelaide

Heaton, R. K. (1981). *Wisconsin Card Sorting Test Manual.* Psychological Assessment Resources, Odessa, Florida

Hechtman, L. (1991). Resilience and vulnerability in long-term outcome of attention deficit disorder. *Canadian Journal of Psychiatry*, 36, pp. 415–21

Helman, C. (1984). *Culture, Health and Illness.* Wright, London

Hill, J. (1996). Letter to the editors. *Journal of Child Psychotherapy*, 22 (2), under Correspondence, pp. 313–15

Hinshaw, S. P. (1994). *Attention Deficits and Hyperactivity in Children.* Sage Publications, London

Hynd, G. W., Semrud-Clikeman, M., Lorys, A. R., Novey, E. S. & Eliopulas, D. (1993). Brain morphology in developmental dyslexia and attention deficit disorder/hyperactivity. *Archives of Neurology*, 47, pp. 919–26

Ingersoll, B. & Goldstein, S. (1993). *Attention Deficit Disorder and Learning Disabilities: Realities, myths and controversial treatments.* Doubleday, New York

Jacobvitz, D., Sroufe, A., Stewart, M. & Leffert, N. (1990). Treatment of attentional and hyperactivity problems in children with sympathomimetic drugs: A comprehensive review. *Journal of the American Academy of Child and Adolescent Psychiatry*, 29, p. 5

James, W. (1980/1981). *The Principles of Psychology.* Harvard University Press, Cambridge, Massachusetts

Jones, C. (1999). Hands-off teaching in the age of mistrust. *The Age*, Melbourne, 4 December, p. 15

Jureidini, J. (2001). Kids & drugs (article by Carmel Sparke). *HQ*, 80, March, pp. 90–5

Kagan, J. (1966). Reflection-impulsivity: The generality and dynamics of conceptual tempo. *Journal of Abnormal Psychology*, 71, pp. 17–24

Kameenui, E. & Simmons, D. (1990). *Designing Instructional Strategies: The prevention of academic and learning problems.* Merrill, Columbus

Kamphaus, R. W., Petoskey, M. & Rowe, E. (2000). Current trends in psychological testing of children. *Professional Psychology, Research and Practice*, 31 (2), pp. 155–64

Kanfer, R. (1992). Work motivation: New directions in theory and research. In C. L. Cooper & I. T. Robertson (eds). *International Review of Industrial and Organizational Psychology*, 7, pp. 1–53

Kaplan, R. M., Sallis, J. S. & Patterson, T. L. (1993). *Health and Human Behaviour*. McGraw-Hill, New York

Karr-Morse, R. & Wiley, M. S. (1997). *Ghosts From the Nursery: Tracing the roots of violence*. The Atlantic Monthly Press, New York

Kellam, S. G., Branch, J. D., Agrawal, K. C., & Ensminger, M. E. (1975). *Mental Health and Going to School, the Woodlawn Program of Assessment, Early Intervention, and Evaluation*. University of Chicago Press, Chicago

Klein, G. L. (1967). Peremptory ideation: Structure and force in motivated ideas. In R. R. Holt (ed.). Motives and thoughts: Psychoanalytic essays in honour of David Rapaport. *Psychological Issues*, 5, pp. 2–3, Monograph 18/19. Referred to in A. J. Sameroff & R. N. Emde (eds). *Relationship Disturbances in Early Childhood*. Basic Books, New York, p. 49

Klein, R. G. & Bessler, A. W. (1992). Stimulant side effects in children. In J. M. Kane and J. A. Lieberman (eds), *Adverse Effects of Psychotropic Drugs*. Guilford Press, New York

Klorman, R. (1991). Cognitive event-related potentials in attention deficit disorder. *Journal of Learning Disabilities*, 24 (3), pp. 130–40

Kohn, A. (1989). Suffer the restless children. *Atlantic Monthly*, November

Kolb, B. (1995). *Brain Plasticity and Behavior*. Lawrence Erlbaum Associates, Mahwah, NJ, USA

Lahat, E., Avital, E., Barr, J., Berkovitch, M., Arlazoroff, A. & Aladjem, M. (1995). BAEP studies in children with attention deficit disorder. *Developmental Medicine and Child Neurology*, 37 (2), pp. 119–23

Lahey, B. B., Applegate, B., McBurnett, K., Greenhill, L., Hynd, G. W., Barkley, R. A., Newcorn, J., Jensen, P. & Richters, J. (1994). DSM field trials for attention deficit hyperactivity disorder in children and adolescents. *American Journal of Psychiatry*, 151, pp. 1673–85

Lahey, B. B., McBurnett, K. & Piacentini, J. C. (1987). Agreement of parent and teacher rating scales with comprehensive clinical assessments of attention deficit disorder with hyperactivity. *Journal of Psychopathology and Behavioral Assessment*, 9, pp. 429–39

Lally, J. R. (1995). The impact of childcare policies and practices on infant/toddler identity formation. *Young Children*, November, pp. 58–67

Leupnitz, D. A. (1988). *The Family Interpreted: Psychoanalysis, feminism, and family therapy*. Basic Books, New York

Levy, F. & Hobbes, G. (1981). The diagnosis of attention deficit disorder (hyperkinesis) in children. *Journal of the American Academy of Child and Adolescent Psychiatry*, 20, pp. 376–84

Lezak, M. D. (1995). *Neuropsychological Assessment* (3rd edn). Wiley, New York

Loeber, R., Green, S. M., Lahey, B. B. & Strouthamer-Loeber, M. (1991). Differences and similarities between children, mothers and teachers as informants on disruptive behaviour disorders. *Journal of Abnormal Child Psychology*, 19, pp. 75–95

Luria, A. R. (1961). *The Role of Speech in the Regulation of Normal and Abnormal Behavior* (J. Tizard ed.). Liveright, New York

Lyon, G. R. & Krasnegor, N. A. (1996). *Attention, Memory and Executive Function*. Paul H. Brookes Publishing Co, Baltimore

McCubbin, M. & Cohen, D. (1999). Empirical, ethical and political perspectives on the use of methylphenidate. *Ethical Human Sciences and Services*. 1 (1), pp. 81–101

McFadyen, A. (1997). Reactivity or hyperactivity. Putting ADHD in a developmental and social context. Talk given at Tavistock Clinic, London. Audiocassette available from Tavistock & Portman, NHS Trust, London, NW 3 5BA, England

McGurk, H. (1997). Human services: changing language—changing concepts? *Family Matters*, 47, pp. 3–4

McGurk, H., Caplan, M., Hennessy, E. & Moss, P. (1993). Controversy, theory and social context in contemporary day care research. *Journal of Child Psychology and Psychiatry*, 34 (1), pp. 3–23

McIntosh, J. (1997). *Promoting Well Being in Child Development: A review of recent literature research and practices*. Victorian Health Promotion Foundation, Issues Series

McKeown, T. (1976). *The Role of Medicine*. Nuffield Provincial Hospitals Trust, London

Mackay, H. (1998). Childhood's brave new world. *The Age*, Melbourne, 8 August, p. 8

Mackey, P. & Kopras, A. (2001). *Medication for Attention Deficit/Hyperactivity Disorder (ADHD): An analysis by Federal electorate.* Current Issues Brief, No. 11 2000–01, Department of the Parliamentary Library, Information and Research Services, Canberra, pp. 1–15

Mahler, M. (1985). *The Psychological Birth of the Human Infant.* Mahler Research Foundation Library, Franklin Lakes, NJ. Videocassette

Main, M., Kaplan, N. & Cassidy, J. (1985). Security in infancy, childhood and adulthood. In I. Bretherton & E. Waters. Growing Points of Attachment Theory and Research. *Monographs of the Society for Research in Child Development,* 209 (50), pp. 66–104

Manly, T., Robertson, I., Anderson, V. & Nimmo-Smith, I. (1999). *Test of Everyday Attention in Children.* Thames Valley Test Company, Cambridge

Mann, E. M., Ikeda, Y., Mueller, C. W., Takahashi, A., Tao, K. T., Humris, E. et al. (1992). Cross-cultural differences in rating hyperactive-disruptive behaviours in children. *American Journal of Psychiatry,* 149 (11), pp. 1539–42

Mannuzza, S., Klein, R. G. & Bessler, A. (1993). Adult outcome of hyperactive boys. Educational achievement, occupational rank, and psychiatric status. *Archives of General Psychiatry,* 42, pp. 937–47

Marris, P. (1986). *Loss and Change.* Revised edn. Routledge & Kegan Paul, London

Mash, E. & Johnstone, C. (1983). Parental perceptions of child behaviour problems, parenting self esteem and mothers' reported stress in younger and older hyperactive and normal children. *Journal of Consulting and Clinical Psychology.* 51, pp. 86–100

Maton, K. J. (2000). Making a difference: The social ecology of social transformation. *American Journal of Community Psychology,* 28 (1), pp. 25–57

Mellor, D. J., Storer, S. P. & Brown, J. (1996). The politics of ADHD. *Australian Educational and Developmental Psychologist,* 13, pp. 40–45

Merrow, J. (1995). ADD—the dubious diagnosis. Public Broadcasting Service, 5 November

Milberger, S., Biederman, J., Faraone, S. V., Chen, L. & Jones, J. (1996). ADHD is associated with early initiation of cigarette smoking in children and adolescents. *Journal of the American Academy of Child and Adolescent Psychiatry,* 36, pp. 37–44

Miller, L., Rustin, M. & Shuttleworth, J. (1989). *Closely Observed Infants.* Duckworth, London

Mirsky, A. F. (1995). Perils and pitfalls on the path to normal potential: The role of impaired attention. *Journal of Clinical and Experimental Neuropsychology*, 17 (4), pp. 481–98

Mirsky, A., Anthony, B., Duncan, C., Ahearn, M. & Kellam, S. (1991). Analysis of the elements of attention: A neuropsychological approach. *Neuropsychological Review*, 2, pp. 109–45

—— (1996). Disorders of attention: A neuropsychological perspective. In G. R. Lyon & N. A. Krasnegor (eds). *Attention, Memory and Executive Function*, Paul H. Brookes Publishing Co., Baltimore, pp. 71–96

Mitchell, B. (1995). Attention deficit disorder 'over-diagnosed'. *The Sunday Age*, Melbourne, 24 September, under News, p. 4

Mosier, C. E. & Rogoff, B. (1994). Infants' instrumental use of their mothers to achieve their goals. *Child Development*, 65 (1), pp. 70–79

Murray, L. (1992). The impact of post natal depression on infant development. *Journal of Child Psychology and Psychiatry*, 133 (3), pp. 543–61

—— (1995). Children's perceptions of family life revealed in doll's house play. Paper presented to conference on New Developments in Attachment Theory—Implications for Adoption and Fostering, at Thomas Coram Foundation, London, England on 30 November

Murray, L. & Trevarthen, C. (1986). The infant's role in mother–infant communications. *Journal of Child Language*, 13, pp. 15–29

Mustard, F. J. & McCain, N. M. (1999). *Reversing the Real Brain Drain: Early Years Study Final Report*. Ontario Children's Secretariat, Publications Ontario, Toronto, Canada

Myers, R. (1992/1995). *The Twelve Who Survive: Strengthening Programmes of Early Childhood Development in the Third World*. High/Scope Press Ypsilanti, Michigan

National Health and Medical Research Council (1997). Attention Deficit Hyperactivity Disorder (ADHD): National Health and Medical Research Council. <*http://www.health.gov.au/nhmrc/publicat/adhd/terms.htm*>

National Institute of Health (1998). Diagnosis and treatment of Attention Deficit Hyperactivity Disorder. NIH Consensus Statement, 16 (2), pp. 1–37

Ncayiyana, D. (1995). *The New Public Health and WHO's Ninth General Programme of Work. A Discussion Paper*. WHO, Division of Development of Human Resources for Health, Geneva

Needleman, H. L., Schell, A., Bellinger, D., Leviton, A. & Allred, E. (1990). The long-term effects of exposure to low doses of lead in childhood. An 11-year follow-up report. *New England Journal of Medicine*, 322 (2), pp. 83–8

New Zealand Ministry of Health (2001). *New Zealand Guidelines for the Assessment and Treatment of Attention Deficit Hyperactivity Disorder.* Ministry of Health, Wellington

Nisbett, R. E. & Ross, L. (1980). *Human Inference: Strategies and shortcomings of social judgement.* Prentice-Hall, Englewood Cliffs, NJ

Ochiltree, G. & Edgar, D. (1995). *Today's Childcare, Tomorrow's Children!* Australian Institute of Family Studies, Melbourne

Papousek, H. & Papousek, M. (1979). Early ontogeny of human social interaction: Its biological roots and social dimensions. In M. von Cranach, K. Foppa, W. Lepenies & D. Ploog (eds). *Human Ethology: Claims and limits of a new discipline.* Cambridge University Press, New York. Referred to in A. J. Sameroff & R. N. Emde (eds). *Relationship Disturbances in Early Childhood.* Basic Books, New York, p. 39

Peloquin, L. J. & Klorman, R. (1986). Effects of methylphenidate on normal children's mood, event related potentials, and performance in memory scanning and vigilance. *Journal of Abnormal Psychology*, 95, pp. 88–9

Perrin, S. & Last, C. G. (1992). Do childhood anxiety measures measure anxiety? *Journal of Abnormal Child Psychology*, 20 (6), pp. 567–78

Perry, B., Pollard, R., Blackley, T., Barker, W. & Vigilante, D. (1995). Childhood trauma, the neurobiology of adaptation and 'use dependent' development of the brain: How 'states' become 'traits'. *Infant Mental Health Journal*, 16 (4), p. 271

Plante, E. & Turkstra, L. (1991). Sources of error in the quantitative analysis of MRI scans. *Magnetic Resonance Imaging*, 9, pp. 589–95

Pless, I. B., Taylor, H. G. & Arsenault, L. (1995). The relationship between vigilance deficits and traffic injuries involving children. *Pediatrics*, 95 (2), pp. 219–24

Polakow, V. (1992). *The Erosion of Childhood* (rev. edn). University of Chicago Press, Chicago

Posner, M. I. (1988). Structures and functions of selective attention. In T. Boll & B. Bryant (eds). *Clinical Neuropsychology and Brain Function: Research, measurement, and practice.* American Psychological Association, pp. 173–201

Power, T. J. (1992). Contextual factors in vigilance testing of children with ADHD. *Journal of Abnormal Child Psychology*, 20, pp. 579–93

Prendergast, M., Taylor, E., Rapoport, J. L., Bartko, J., Donnelly, M., Zametkin, A. et al. (1988). The diagnosis of childhood hyperactivity: A US–UK cross national study of DSM-III and ICD 9. *Journal of Child Psychology and Psychiatry*, 29, pp. 289–300

Prifitera, A. & Desh, J. (1993). Base rates of WISC-III diagnostic subtest patterns among normal, learning disabled, and ADHD samples. In B. A. Bracken & R. S. McCallum (eds). *Journal of Psychoeducational Assessment Monograph Series, Advances in Psychoeducational Assessment: Wechsler Intelligence Scale for Children* (3rd edn). Psychoeducational Corporation, Germantown, TN, pp. 43–55

Prilleltensky, I., Nelson, G. & Peirson, L. (eds). (2001). *Promoting Family Wellness and Preventing Child Maltreatment: Fundamentals for thinking and action*. University of Toronto Press, Toronto.

Prosser, B. (1997). Why ADHD needs urgent attention. *Education Review*, 1 (7), p. 12

—— (1999). Who is responsible for Attention Deficit Hyperactivity Disorder? A critical introduction to policy in South Australia. *Teaching and Teachers' Work*, 7 (1), pp. 1–10

Prosser, B. & Reid, R. (1999). Psychostimulant use for children with ADHD in Australia. *Journal of Emotional and Behavioral Disorders*, 7 (2), pp. 110–17

Psychological Corporation (1996). *Vigil Continuous Performance Test*. San Antonio, TX

Pugh, G. & De'ath, E. (1984). *The Needs of Parents*. National Children's Bureau Series. London

Rapoport, J. L., Buchsbaum, M. S., Zahn, T. P. et al. (1978). Dextroamphetamine: Cognitive and behavioural effects in normal and prepubertal boys. *Science*, 199, pp. 560–3

Rapport, M. D., Denney, C., DuPaul, G. J. & Gardner, M. J. (1994). Attention Deficit Disorder and methylphenidate: Normalization rates, clinical effectiveness, and response prediction in 76 children. *Journal of the American Academy of Child and Adolescent Psychiatry*, 32, pp. 333–42

Reid, R. (1995) Assessment of ADHD with culturally different groups: The use of behavioural rating scales. *School Psychology Review*, 24, 4, pp. 537–60

Reid, R., Maag, J. W. & Vasa, S. F. (1993). Attention Deficit Hyperactivity Disorder as a disability category: A critique. *Exceptional Children*, 60, pp. 198–214

Riccio, C. A., Reynolds, C. R. & Lowe, P. A. (2001). *Clinical applications of Continuous Performance Tests: Measuring attention and impulsive responding in children and adults.* Wiley, New York

Richman, M., Stevenson, J. & Graham, P. J. (1982). *Pre-school to School: A behavioural study.* Academic Press, London

Rie, H., Rie, E., Stewart, S. & Anbuel, J. (1976). Effects of Ritalin on underachieving children: A replication. *American Journal of Orthopsychiatry,* 45 (2), pp. 313–22

Robertson, J. (1989). *Separation and the Very Young.* Free Association Books, London

Rosenhan, D. L. (1973). On being sane in insane places. *Science,* 179, pp. 250–8

Rosenhan, D. L. (1984). On being sane in insane places. Reprinted in Paul Watzlawick (ed). *The Invented Reality.* WW Norton & Co., New York

Rowe K. J. & Rowe, K. S. (1995). *The Rowe Behavioural Rating Inventory User's Manual. Teacher and parent administered inventories for the assessment of child externalising behaviours for use in clinical, educational and epidemiological research.* Centre for Applied Educational Research, The University of Melbourne, Melbourne

Rueckert, L. & Grafman, L. (1996). Sustained attention in patients with right frontal lesions. *Neuropsychologia,* 34, pp. 953–63

Rutter, M. (1978). Family, area and school influences in the genesis of conduct disorders. In L. A. Hersov & D. Schaffer (eds). *Aggression and Anti-Social Behaviour in Childhood and Adolescence.* Pergamon Press, Oxford, pp. 95–114

—— (1982). Syndrome attributed to minimal brain dysfunction. *Journal of Psychiatry,* 139, pp. 21–33

—— (1990). Psychosocial resilience and protective mechanisms. In J. Rolf, A. S. Masten, D. Cicchetti, K. H. Nuechterlein & S. Weintraub. *Risk and Protective Factors in the Development of Psychopathology.* Cambridge University Press, Cambridge, pp. 181–214

Rutter, M. & Smith D. (eds) (1995). *Psychosocial Disorders in Young People.* Wiley, Chichester

Rutter, M., Tizard, J. & Whitmore, K. (1970). *Eduational Health and Behaviour.* Longmans, London

Safran, J. S. & Safran, S. P. (1987). Teachers' judgments of problem behaviors. *Exceptional Children,* 54, pp. 240–4

Sameroff, A. J. & Emde, R. N. (eds) (1989). *Relationship Disturbances in Early Childhood.* Basic Books, New York

Sanson, A., Smart, D., Prior, M. & Oberklaid, F. (1993). Precursors of hyperactivity and aggression. *Journal of the American Academy of Child and Adolescent Psychiatry*, 32, pp. 1207–16

Sawyer, M. et al. (2000). *Mental Health of Young People in Australia*, Department of Health and Aged Care, Canberra

Schachar, R., Sandberg, S. & Rutter, M. (1986). Agreement between teacher ratings and observations of hyperactivity, inattentiveness and defiance. *Journal of Abnormal Child Psychology*, 14, pp. 331–45

Schmidt Neven, R. (1994). *Exploring Parenthood: A psychodynamic approach for a changing society.* Australian Council for Educational Research, Melbourne

—— (1995). Developing a psychotherapy clinic for children, parents and young people at a large paediatric hospital in Australia. *Journal of Child Psychotherapy*, 21 (1), pp. 91–120

—— (1996). *Emotional Milestones: From birth to adulthood—a psychodynamic approach.* Australian Council for Educational Research, Melbourne

Schmuck, R. A. & Schmuck, P. A. (1983). *Group Processes in the Classroom.* Wm. C. Brown Company Publishers, Dubuque, Iowa

Schore, A. N. (1994). *Affect Regulation and the Origin of Self.* Erlbaum, Hillsdale, NJ

—— (1996). The experience-dependent maturation of a regulatory system in the orbital prefrontal cortex and the origin of developmental psychopathology. *Development and Psychopathology*, 8, pp. 59–87

Schwartz, G. E. (1982). Testing the biopsychosocial model: The ultimate challenge facing behavioral medicine? *Journal of Consulting and Clinical Psychology*, 50, pp. 1040–53

Sergeant, J. (1996). A theory of attention: An information processing perspective. In G. R. Lyon & N. A. Krasnegor (eds). *Attention, Memory, and Executive Function.* Paul Brooks Publishing Co., Baltimore, pp. 57–69

Shaffer, D. (1994). Attention deficit hyperactivity disorder in adults. *American Journal of Psychiatry*, 151, pp. 633–8

Shaw, D. S. et al. (1996). Early risk factors and pathways in the development of early disruptive behaviour problems. *Development and Psychopathology*, 8, pp. 679–99

Shaw, D. W. & Vondra, J. I. (1995). Infant attachment security and maternal predictors of early behaviour problems. A longitudinal study of low-income families. *Journal of Abnormal Child Psychology*, 23, pp. 335–57

Shaywitz, B. A. & Shaywitz, S. E. (1991). Comorbidity: A critical issue in attention deficit disorder. *Journal of Child Neurology*, 6, Suppl: S13–22

Shaywitz, S. E., Fletcher, J. M. & Shaywitz, B. A. (1994). Issues in the definition and classification of attention deficit disorder. *Topics in Language Disorders*, 14 (4), pp. 1–25

Shenker, A. (1992). The mechanism of action of drugs used to treat attention deficit hyperactivity disorder: Focus on catecholamine receptor pharmacology. *Advances in Pediatrics*, 39, pp. 337–82

Shiffrin, R. M & Schneider, W. (1977). Controlled and automatic human information processing: II. Perceptual learning, automatic attending, and a general theory. *Psychological Review*, 84, pp. 127–90

Shine, K. (2001). Toddlers prescribed drugs for behaviour. *Sunday Age News*, Melbourne, 18 February

Shore, R. (1997). *Rethinking the Brain: New insights into early development*. Families and Work Institute, New York

Shukla, V. K. & Otten, N. (1999). Assessment of ADHD therapy. A Canadian perspective. *CCOHTA*. January

Siegel, D. J. (2001). Toward an interpersonal neurobiology of the developing mind: Attachment relationships, 'mindsight', and neural integration. *Infant Mental Health Journal*, 22 (1–2), pp. 67–94

Sinason, V. (1992). *Mental Handicap and the Human Condition*. Free Association Books, London

Sivanandan, A. (1994). Behaviour problems. In J. Bourne, L. Bridges & C. Searle (eds). *Outcast England: How schools exclude black children*. Institute of Race Relations, London

Skynner, R. (1996) *Family Matters: A guide to healthier and happier relationships*. Cedar, London

Smith, D. (1995). Youth crime and conduct disorders: Trends, patterns and causal explanations. In M. Rutter & D. Smith (eds). *Psychosocial Disorders in Young People*. Wiley, Chichester. Referred to in P. Cooper (1998). Developments in the Understanding of Childhood Emotional and Behavioural Problems Since 1981. In R. Laslett, P. Cooper, P. Maras, A. Rimmer & A. Law (eds). *Changing Perceptions: Emotional and behavioural difficulties since 1945*. The Association of Workers for Children with Emotional and Behavioural Difficulties, Kent, p. 43

Snow, C. E. (1972). Mother's speech to children learning language. *Child Development*, 43, pp. 549–65. Referred to in A. J. Sameroff

& R. N. Emde (eds). *Relationship Disturbances in Early Childhood.* Basic Books, New York, p. 39

Sohlberg, M. M. & Mateer, C. A. (2001). *Cognitive Rehabilitation: An integrative neuropsychological approach.* Guilford Press, New York

Sonuga-Barke, E. J., Houlberg, K. & Hall, M. (1994). When is impulsiveness not impulsive? The case of the hyperactive children's cognitive style. *Journal of Child Psychology and Psychiatry and Allied Disciplines,* 35 (7), pp. 1247–53

Sonuga-Barke, E. J. S., Minocha, K., Taylor, E. A. & Sandberg, S. (1993). Inter-ethnic bias in teachers' ratings of childhood - hyperactivity. *British Journal of Developmental Psychology,* 11, pp. 187–200

Spencer, T. J., Biederman, J. & Wilens, T. (1998). Pharmacotherapy with antidepressants. In R. A. Barkley, *Attention Deficit Disorder: A handbook for diagnosis and treatment* (2nd edn). Guilford Press, New York

Sroufe, L. A. (1989). *Relationships and Relationship Disturbances.* Referred to in A. J. Sameroff & R. N. Emde (eds). *Relationship Disturbances in Early Childhood.* Basic Books, New York, p. 82

Sroufe, L. A. & Waters, E. (1977). Attachment as an organisational construct. *Child Development,* 48, pp. 1184–99

Stadtler, Ann C. et al. (1995). The Touchpoints Model: Building supportive alliances between parents and professionals. *Zero to Three,* August/September

Stern, D. N. (1977). *The First Relationship: Infant and mother.* Harvard Uni. Press, Cambridge

—— (1985). *The Interpersonal World of the Infant: A view from psychoanalysis and developmental psychology.* Basic Books, New York

Stevens, G. (1981). Bias in the attribution of hyperkinetic behavior as a function of ethnic identification and socioeconomic status. *Psychology in the Schools,* 18, pp. 99–106

Stiefel, I. (1997). Can disturbance in attachment contribute to Attention Deficit Hyperactivity Disorder? A case discussion. *Clinical Child Psychology and Psychiatry,* 2 (1), pp. 45–64

Still, G. F. (1902). Some abnormal psychiatric conditions in children. *Lancet,* I, pp. 1008–12, pp. 1077–82, pp. 1163–68. Referred to in The British Psychological Society (1996). *Attention Deficit Hyperactivity Disorder (ADHD): A psychological response to an evolving concept,* p. 13

Strean, H. S. (1997). Who is father? Where is father? Some facts, fantasies and fallacies. *Journal of Analytic Social Work*, 4 (3), pp. 5–22

Streissguth, A. P., Sampson, P. D., Carmichael Oldon, H., Bookstein, F. L., Barr, H. M., Scott, M., Feldman, J. & Mirsky, A. F. (1994). Maternal drinking during pregnancy: Attention and short-term memory performance in 14-year-old offspring: A longitudinal prospective study. *Alcoholism: Clinical and Experimental Research*, 18, pp. 202–18

Stuss, D. & Benson, D. F. (1984). Neuropsychological studies of the frontal lobes. *Psychological Bulletin*, 95, pp. 3–28

Svigos, G. (1998). Drugs a quick-fix for problem kids. *Progress Press*, Melbourne, 17 August, p. 7

Swanson, J. M., Lerner, M. & Williams, L. (1995). More frequent diagnosis of attention deficit-hyperactivity disorder. *The New England Journal of Medicine*, 333, p. 944

Swanson, J. M., McBurnett, K., Wigal, T., Pfifner, L. J. et al. (1993). Effect of stimulant medication on children with attention deficit disorder: A 'review of reviews'. *Exceptional Children*, 60, 2, pp. 154–62

Szatmari, P., Offord, D. R. & Boyle, M. H. (1989). Ontario child health study: Prevalence of attention deficit disorder with hyperactivity. *Journal of Child Psychology and Psychiatry*, 30, pp. 219–30

Szaz, T. (1961). *Ideology and Insanity: Essays on the psychiatric dehumanization of man*. Syracuse University Press, Syracuse, NY

Szur, R. & Miller, S. (eds) (1991). *Extending Horizons: Psychoanalytic psychotherapy with children, adolescents and families*. Karnac Books, London

Taylor, E. & Hemsley, R. (1995). Treating hyperkinetic disorders in children. *British Medical Journal*, 310, pp. 1617–18

Taylor, H. (1988). Learning disabilities. In E. Mash (ed.). *Behavioral Assessments of Childhood Disorders*. Guilford Press, New York, pp. 402–5

Thomas, J. M., Benham, A. L., Gean, M., Luby, J., Minde, K., Turner, S. & Wright, H. H. (1997). Practice parameters for the psychiatric assessment of infants and toddlers (0–36 months). *Journal of the American Academy of Child and Adolescent Psychiatry*, 36, pp. 218–368

Thompson, R. F. & Bettinger, L. A. (1970). Neural substrates of attention. In D. I. Mostofsky (ed.). *Attention: Contemporary theory and analysis*. Appleton-Century-Crofts, New York, pp. 367–401

Tracey, N. (1993). *Mothers, Fathers Speak on the Drama of Pregnancy, Birth and the First Year of Life.* Apollo Books, London

Trevarthen, C. (1979). Communication and cooperation in early infancy: A description of primary intersubjectivity. In M. Bullowa (ed.). *Before speech: The beginnings of communication.* Cambridge University Press, Cambridge

—— (1986). In L. Murray & C. Trevarthen. The infant's role in mother–infant communications. *Journal of Child Language,* 13, pp. 15–29

—— (2001). Intrinsic motives for companionship in understanding: Their origin, development, and significance for infant mental health. *Infant Mental Health Journal.* 22 (1–2), pp. 95–131

Trowell, J. (ed.) (1995). *The Emotional Needs of Young Children and Their Families.* Routledge, London

Tulchin, T. H. & Varavikova, E. A. (2000). *The New Public Health— An introduction for the 21st century.* Academic Press, San Diego

Ullman, R. K. & Sleator, E. K. (1986). Responders, nonresponders and placebo responders among others during a treatment evaluation. *Clinical Pediatrics,* 25, pp. 594–99

United States Drug Enforcement Administration (1995). *Methylphenidate.* US Department of Justice, Drug and Chemical Evaluation Section Office of Diversion Control, Arlington, Virginia

Uzgiris, I. (1976). *Organisation and Sensorimotor Intelligence.* Plenum, New York

Valentine, J., Zubrick, S. & Sly, P. (1996). National trends in the use of stimulant medication for attention deficit disorder. *Journal of Paediatrics and Child Health,* 32 (3), pp. 223–7

Vandell, D. L. & Corasaniti, M. A. (1990). Variations in early child care: Do they predict subsequent social, emotional and cognitive differences? *Early Childhood Research Quarterly,* 5, pp. 555–72

Van der Kolk, B. (1998) The psychology and psychobiology of developmental trauma. In A. Stoudemire (ed.) *Human Behaviour: An introduction for medical students.* Lippincott-Raven, New York

Van Zomeren, A. H. & Brouwer, W. H. (1994). *Clinical Neuropsychology of Attention.* Oxford University Press, New York

Vygotsky, L. S. (1962). *Thought and Language.* Wiley, New York

Wakefield, J. C. (1992). The concept of mental disorder: On the boundary between biological facts and social values. *American Psychologist,* 47, pp. 373–88

Walker, K. (1999). Ensuring that early childhood practices and programs reflect current research and knowledge in child development. Paper presented at the Australian Early Childhood Association National Conference, Darwin, July 1999

Ward, S. (1995). Article in *The Guardian* newspaper, August

—— (2000). *Baby Talk*. Century, UK

Wechsler, D. (1991). *WISC-III Manual*. The Psychological Corporation, San Antonio, TX

Weinberg, W. A. & Brumback, R. A. (1992). The myth of attention deficit-hyperactivity disorder: Symptoms resulting from multiple causes. *Journal of Child Neurology*, 7, pp. 431–5

Weinberg, W. A. & Emslie, G. J. (1991). Attention Deficit Hyperactivity Disorder: The differential diagnosis. *Journal of Child Neurology*, 6, Suppl. S23–36

Weinstein, C. (1994). Cognitive remediation strategies. *Journal of Psychotherapy Practice and Research*. 3 (1), pp. 44–57

Weiss, G. & Hechtman, L. (1993). *Hyperactive Children Grown Up*. Guilford Press, New York

Weiss, R. E., Stein, M. A., Trommer, B. & Refetoff, S. (1993). Attention deficit hyperactivity disorder and thyroid function. *Journal of Pediatrics*, 123 (4), pp. 539–45

Whalen, C. K. & Henker, B. (1996) Attention Deficit/Hyperactivity Disorders. In T. H. Ollendick and M. Hersen (eds). *Handbook of Child Psychopathology* (3rd edn). Plenum Press, New York

Whalen, C. K., Henker, B., Collins, B. E., Finck, D. & Dotemoto, S. (1979). A social ecology of hyperactive boys: Medication effects in systematically structured classroom environments. *Journal of Applied Behavioral Analysis*, 12, pp. 65–81

Whitehead, W.E., Busch, C. M., Heller, B. R. & Costa, P. T. (1986). Social learning influences on menstrual symptoms and illness behavior. *Health Psychology*, 5, pp. 13–23

WHO (World Health Organization) (1993). *International Classification of Diseases.* 10th revision (ICD-10). Classification of Mental and Behavioural Disorders. Diagnostic Criteria for Research. WHO, Geneva

Widener, A, J. (1998). Beyond Ritalin: The importance of therapeutic work with parents and children diagnosed ADD/ADHD. *Journal of Child Psychotherapy*, 24 (2), pp. 267–81

Wielkiewicz, R. M. (1990). Interpreting low scores on the WISC-R Third factor: It's more than distractibility. *Psychological Assessment: Journal of Consulting and Clinical Psychology*, 2 (1), pp. 91–7

Wilson, E. O. (1998). *Consilience: The unity of knowledge*. Vintage, New York

Winnicott, D. W. (1947). Hate in the countertransference. In Dodi Goldman (ed.). *In One's Bones: The clinical genius of Winnicott*. (1993). Jason Aronson Inc

—— (1958). Primary maternal preoccupation. In *Collected Papers: Through paediatrics to psychoanalysis*. Tavistock, London

—— (1964). *The Child, the Family and the Outside World*. Penguin Books, Harmondsworth

—— (1965a). The capacity to be alone. In *The Maturational Processes and the Facilitating Environment*. Hogarth Press, London

—— (1965b). The theory of the parent infant relationship. In *The Maturational Processes and the Facilitating Environment*. Hogarth Press, London

—— (1971). *Playing and Reality*. Penguin, Harmondsworth

—— (1988). *Babies and their Mothers*. Free Association Books, London

Wolraich, M. L., Lindgren, S. & Stromquist, A. (1990). Stimulant medication use by primary care physicians in the treatment of attention deficit hyperactivity disorder. *Pediatrics*, 86, pp. 95–101

Yelich, G. & Salamone, F. (1994). Constructivist interpretation of Attention Deficit Hyperactivity Disorder. *Journal of Constructivist Psychology*, 7, pp. 191–212

Young Minds (1999a). American children with ADHD are receiving inconsistent care. 38, January–February, news item pp. 4–5

—— (1999b). NHS prescriptions of Ritalin double in 12 months. 38, January–February, news item p. 8

—— (2000). Prescribing Ritalin to all who could benefit would cost 44 million pounds. 49, November–December, news item p. 5

Zametkin, A. J., Liebenauer, L. L., Fitzgerald, G. A., King, A. C., Minkunas, D. V., Herscovitch, P., Yamada, E. M. & Cohen, R. M. (1993). Brain metabolism in teenagers with attention deficit hyperactivity disorder. *Archives of General Psychiatry*, 50 (5), pp. 333–40

Zametkin, A. J., Nordahl, T. E., Gross, M., King, A. C., Semple, W. E., Rumsey, J., Hamburger, S. & Cohen, R. (1990). Cerebral glucose metabolism in adults with hyperactivity of childhood onset. *New England Journal of Medicine*, 323, pp. 1361–6

Zentall, S. (1975). Optimal stimulation as a theoretical basis of hyperactivity. *American Journal of Orthopsychiatry*, 45, pp. 549–61

Index

Page numbers in bold type, e.g. **16–21** indicate detailed discussion of the topic.

The Centre for Child and Family Development

The Centre promotes awareness and understanding of the emotional life of children and adolescents and how this affects their behaviour and future development. The centre offers:

- The psychotherapy clinic for children, parents and young peoples
- Professional training and supervision
- Organisational and consulting services
- Exploring Parenthood workshops and talks

The Centre for Child and Family Development
721a Riversdale Road
Camberwell
Victoria 3124
Tel 03 9830 0422
Tax 03 9830 0455
Email ccfdau@ozemail.com.au
www.childandfamily.com.au